NURSING THEORY

Analysis • Application • Evaluation

Fifth Edition

DATE DUE

OCT 1 9 1998	
NOV 2 4 1998	
APR 2 1 1999	
SEP 27 1999	
APR 1 9 2002	
OCT - 6 2003	

BRODART   Cat. No. 23-221

NURSING THEORY
Analysis · Application · Evaluation
Fifth Edition

Barbara Stevens Barnum, RN, PhD, FAAN
Professor of Clinical Nursing
Columbia University School of Nursing
New York, New York

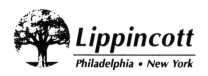 **Lippincott**
Philadelphia · New York

Acquisitions Editor: Susan M. Glover, RN, MSN
Assistant Editor: Bridget Blatteau
Project Editor: Gretchen Metzger
Senior Production Manager: Helen Ewan
Production Coordinator: Patricia McCloskey
Design Coordinator: Nicholas Rook
Indexer: Victoria Boyle

Edition 5

9 8 7 6 5 4 3 2 1

Library of Congress Cataloging-in-Publication Data

Barnum, Barbara Stevens.
    Nursing theory : analysis, application, evaluation / Barbara
Stevens Barnum. — 5th ed.
        p.   cm.
    Includes bibliographical references and index.
    ISBN 0-7817-1104-5 (alk. paper)
    1. Nursing—Philosophy.   I. Title.
    [DNLM: 1. Nursing Theory.   WY 86 B263n 1998]
TR84.5.B37   1998
610.73'01—dc21
DNLM/DLC
for Library of Congress   97-30274
                                                                CIP

Care has been taken to confirm the accuracy of the information presented and to describe generally accepted practices. However, the authors, editors, and publisher are not responsible for errors or omissions or for any consequences from application of the information in this book and make no warranty, express or implied, with respect to the contents of the publication.

The authors, editors, and publisher have exerted every effort to ensure that drug selection and dosage set forth in this text are in accordance with current recommendations and practice at the time of publication. However, in view of ongoing research, changes in government regulations, and the constant flow of information relating to drug therapy and drug reactions, the reader is urged to check the package insert for each drug for any change in indications and dosage and for added warnings and precautions. This is particularly important when the recommended agent is a new or infrequently employed drug.

Some drugs and medical devices presented in this publication have Food and Drug Administration (FDA) clearance for limited use in restricted research settings. It is the responsibility of the health care provider to ascertain the FDA status of each drug or device planned for use in their clinical practice.

For Donald G. Fern

*With gratitude
for the many weekends you spent alone
without complaining,
while I gave the computer my full attention
in completing this 5th edition.*

Reviewers

Mary Ann Hautman, RN, PhD
Professor
School of Nursing
University of San Diego
San Diego, California

Alice S. Hill, RN, PhD
Associate Professor
School of Nursing
The University of Texas Medical Branch
Galveston, Texas

Daniel J. Pesut, PhD, RN, CS, FAAN
Associate Professor
College of Nursing
University of South Carolina
Columbia, South Carolina

Barbara A. Vellenga, PhD, RN
Professor
Nursing Department
Moorhead State University
Moorehead, Minnesota

Preface to the Fifth Edition

In many ways, nursing theory has changed radically since the past edition of *Nursing Theory: Analysis, Application, Evaluation.* These changes reflect the changing worlds of nursing practice and nursing education. Chief among these changes is the nationwide movement to managed care, moving nursing theory toward an outcomes orientation. The radical expansion of clinical sites for care delivery beyond the acute care hospital has moved theory in two directions: (1) theory as extracted from the delivery setting, and (2) theory as environment dependent. Reduced resources in both care facilities and schools have further impacted on nursing theory by making goals, particularly economic ones, increasingly important in theoretical models. Additionally, the rapid growth of the nurse practitioner movement has led to a theory focus on roles, and increased sophistication in nursing research has caused a greater focus on middle-range theory because concepts at this level are more capable of being tested by research.

These trends represent only a few of those affecting nursing theory today. In an era when change is fast-coming on many fronts, it is not surprising that theory is often tentative and incompletely developed. It is also not surprising that many writers focus on process rather than content elements, with the hope that the processes will last even if the content changes. The focus on critical thinking illustrates this point, with this notion inserted in many newer theories.

It is an exciting time to be associated with nursing, despite its stresses, and it is a fascinating time in which to consider nursing theory. Some of my graduate students whose earlier theory courses were composed of reviews of the early "grand" theorists initially have difficulty seeing nursing theory as a vital component of their education. Most change their minds by the end of the term, for theory does much more than review past efforts. A good theory course teaches students to think, to question everything they read, to understand when an argument is valid or invalid, and to know that it is better to act out of knowledge than out of ignorance.

The reader will find examples of the *new* environment of nursing, but in other ways, this book is unchanged. The purpose has always been to teach students to think and conceptualize within their chosen profession, and many things do not change: how to follow an argument, how to determine the logic of a position, or how to evaluate a proposal. For readers who wish to learn to *think* while they study theory, the fifth edition will continue to provide that direction.

Barbara Stevens Barnum, RN, PhD, FAAN

Preface to the Fourth Edition

Nursing theory has changed in many ways since the first edition of this book. No longer a strange concept, nursing theory is now discussed in hundreds of books and journals. Extant theories are no longer limited in number but have proliferated on all levels—grand, middle range, and narrow range. Unlike many disciplines, the profession of nursing seems satisfied with a proliferation of conceptual frameworks, though various approaches wax and wane in popularity.

For the student of theory, *Nursing Theory: Analysis, Application, Evaluation, Fourth Edition* provides the tools for understanding, analyzing, and evaluating nursing theories. Although most of the popular theories are illustrated and discussed, the book is not intended to serve as a comprehensive survey of theories. Instead, the book should be used along with original works on theory. The reader is strongly encouraged to reach original theory formulations rather than secondary interpretations of them, which may or may not be accurate. This book, then, is a work of metatheory—about theory—not a nursing theory itself. *The only intent is to prepare the user to read theory with comprehension.*

This edition, like the previous editions, takes primarily an analytic viewpoint, that is, looking at what has been written about nursing theory and subjecting the writing to semantic analysis. One cannot effectively analyze a theorist—she is a moving target—but one can analyze a given piece of writing.

In this text numerous theory works have been drawn upon to illustrate points of analysis. The reader should not expect that the examples necessarily represent the most recent work of a theorist. Instead, they are works that best illustrate a point being made.

In addition to looking at theory writings, nursing practices that have theoretical implications will be examined. Between analyzing what is written and what is done, it is hoped that the reader will come away effective in applying theory-colored glasses to all endeavors of nursing.

Because readers and the vast majority of theorists in nursing are women, the feminine gender has been used throughout this book. The men of our profession are asked once more to show their flexibility and to accept this choice rather than have every reader face the distortions of content and syntax that result from using the non-gendered plural. Theory analysis requires a precision that is often lost when things are stated in the plural.

Finally, the reader will find that the term *theory* is used here to stand for all constructs—paradigms, if you prefer—however complete or tentative in their formulation. People who hold to rigid definitions of what comprises a theory may be uncomfortable with this usage, preferring to reserve the term *theory* for the highest level formulations. Since few theories of nursing have yet reached that pinnacle, I prefer to use the term more liberally, making the point that theory work is important at every level of endeavor.

Barbara J. Stevens Barnum, RN, PhD, FAAN

Acknowledgments

Each edition of *Nursing Theory* has been shaped by reactions from students, never more so than in this 5th edition. The students I presently teach at Columbia University are doctoral or master's degree students, the latter studying to become nurse practitioners. Doctoral students, only a few in each class, provide a wonderful source for discourse on theory and theory-related matters. Yet the master's degree students are my greatest challenge. Most of them are highly immersed in the study of physiology, pathology, and vast quantities of technical information. They are learning to handle independent primary care decision making; they want practical knowledge that applies to their careers. These students descend upon nursing theory courses demanding relevance, application, and immediate utility—from a subject often prejudged as esoteric and relatively unimportant. In one sense they are right; few patients die from application of the wrong nursing theory. In another sense, they are equally wrong; a good theory course should, above all else, teach one to think critically—a skill that comes in handy in any number of situations, nursing included.

It gives me great satisfaction, then, when so many of these students come to appreciate the charms (and benefits) of studying nursing theory. Columbia master's degree students and doctoral students alike inevitably refuse to let me coast on past glories. Their inquisitive minds keep formulating new questions that force me to analyze things in new ways. Hopefully, this new edition of *Nursing Theory* will reflect some of the dialogues in which we have engaged. For this teaching challenge, I thank and acknowledge my students.

I would also like to thank my research assistant, Ms. Joyce Tan Neria, who kept me updated on nursing theory, inundating me with readings—those that I requested and those she thought I shouldn't miss. Without her assistance, I would still be muddling through rewriting the first chapter.

Barbara Stevens Barnum

Contents

1   *What Is Nursing Theory?*

WHAT IS A THEORY?

Not everyone agrees on the meaning of the word *theory*. Some use it only for a complex set of interrelated principles that describe or explain a phenomenon, using other words like *construct* or *conceptual framework* for less developed sets or those with fewer as yet unrelated variables. In this book, we consider such differences to be mere splitting of hairs. For our purposes, a theory will contain both low level and highly developed structures. A theory is a construct that accounts for or organizes some phenomenon. A nursing theory, then, describes or explains nursing. It is a shorthand way to characterize a phenomenon, to point out those components or characteristics that give the phenomenon its identity. Theory pulls out the salient parts, separating the critical and necessary factors (or relationships) from the accidental and unessential factors.

A theory is like a map of a territory as opposed to an aerial photograph. The map does not display the full terrain (buildings, moving vehicles, grazing livestock); instead, it picks out the parts that are important for its purpose. If its aim is to guide travelers, the map will highlight roads; if its purpose is to describe the physical terrain, it shows mountains, plains, and rivers. But no map (or theory) reflects all that is contained within a phenomenon. Such a map would defeat its purpose, that of giving one a handle on the phenomenon. The handle is created by making the essential parts stand out in relief.

Visintainer (1986) uses the map analogy in the following explanation:

> *The maps of a discipline operate in a way similar to that of maps of a geographic region. They provide a framework for selecting and organiz-*

1

ing information from the environment. In studying a discipline, one learns the maps and through mastery of the maps learns what to ask about, what to observe, what to focus on, what to think about. (p. 33)

Different theories of nursing use different maps. That is, diverse components and relationships assume importance in disparate theories. As Visintainer (1986) has noted, "Viewing the world through different maps can produce strange twists to a territory with which we are familiar" (p. 35).

There are at least two different types of theories. Some constructs assert something about the way in which a subject exists; others simply give one way in which the thing may be organized. For example, consider the big bang theory of the universe. This theory proposes something about the creation and subsequent behavior of the universe. It has the potential for being proven or disproved. Similarly, when Einstein's conception of physics replaced Newton's physics, the new theory corrected errors of fact in the older schema.

Theories of nursing are not constructs of this dimension. Instead, they offer alternate ways in which to describe and organize the content of the discipline. One cannot, for example, say that use of the nursing process and nursing diagnoses (a popular modern theory) is *true*, whereas Orem's self-care theory is *false*. Instead, they represent alternate ways to categorize and make sense of nursing phenomena; they are preferences for organizing thought and action, not irrevocable statements about reality.

TYPES OF THEORY

Theories are classified in many different ways, including their level of development. One such classification simply divides them into those that describe and those that explain.

Descriptive Theory

The *descriptive theory* looks at a phenomenon and identifies its major elements or events (relationships among elements). The theory does not, however, say why the phenomenon has those elements or events, how they relate to each other, or how changes in the elements or relations affect each other.

In its simplest form, this theory looks at a phenomenon and names its major constituents (elements or events). This lowest level of description is called *ad hoc theory*. Ad hoc theory looks at the phenomenon—for example, a basket for simplicity—and sees that it contains apples, oranges, and baseballs. It does not explain why baseballs are present with apples and oranges; it merely states that such is the case. Thus, the ad hoc theory is primitive, simply pointing out what exists.

When the constituents of a descriptive theory share some structural interrelationship, the theory is termed *categorical* or *classificatory* rather than *ad hoc*. This is the first effort at sorting what is contained in the theory. Sometimes the relationship among identified elements is one of invariant, logical sequence. The nursing process, for example, uses the principle of logical sequence. Patient assessment must precede and lead to diagnosis; diagnosis then leads to the next step, and so forth until the process is completed.

The relationship among theory parts in a categorical descriptive theory usually is one in which the constituents are mutually exclusive and sometimes exhaustive parts. For example, one nursing theory divides the human being into separate spiritual, physical, and psychological components.

The theories of King and Levine illustrate the difference between ad hoc and categorical descriptions. King (1981, pp. 10–12) builds a conceptual framework with nursing interacting systems based on personal systems, interpersonal systems, and social systems. Because these systems are based on ever-expanding numbers of interactions (individuals, groups, society), this part of the theory can be labeled as categorical. Yet subcomponents under these labels lack this sort of tidy organization. For example, in relation to personal systems, King (1981) had said, "Selected concepts are . . . (1) perception, (2) self, (3) body image, (4) growth and development, (5) time, and (6) space" (p. 10). Obviously these elements are not all one of a kind, so at this level, the theory is ad hoc.

Levine (1971) uses a categorical schema:

> *There are four major areas of care in which nursing can fulfill a conservation function. They are embodied in the conservation principles of nursing:*
>
> 1. *Nursing intervention is based on the conservation of the individual patient's energy.*
> 2. *Nursing intervention is based on the conservation of the individual patient's structural integrity.*
> 3. *Nursing intervention is based on the conservation of the individual patient's personal integrity.*
> 4. *Nursing intervention is based on the conservation of the individual patient's social integrity. (p. 258)*

Clearly, Levine's four conservation principles are mutually exclusive, but it would be more difficult to assert that they are mutually exhaustive components. Someone might come along and think of a fifth component to be added to the model. Notice Levine's symmetry: all four principles are types of conservation.

The descriptive theory represents the *first level* of work in theory development, that is, it identifies the salient constituents of a theory, naming the elements or events. A descriptive theory may point out complex and abstract concepts, but it is not explanatory if it fails to explain why the phenomenon is as it is or acts as it does. A descriptive theory is an existential statement; it asserts *what is.*

Descriptive theory is not only the first level of theory development but the most important because it determines what will be perceived as the essence of the phenomenon under study. Subsequent development of a theory will expand on or refine those elements and relationships selected as salient in the descriptive phase. The course of subsequent theory development is channeled by the initial selection of elements seen as critical.

Because most subsequent work on a theory will go into explaining the described elements or events (even if additional elements are added along the way), it is critical that the most significant constituents be recognized and named. Elements and events are not self-evident, so naming is not merely reiteration of the obvious. Even in our example of the basket of apples, oranges, and baseballs, it would have been possible to characterize the phenomenon in different ways, for example, as a collection of red, orange, and white spheres. Given this characterization of the elements, a basket of red jacks balls, tangerines, and ping-pong balls would be recognized as another instance of the same phenomenon. Yet another description of the basket's contents might characterize them according to size, number, or weights of the elements.

As an exercise in deriving descriptive theory, the reader is invited to see how many different ways our hypothetical basket could be characterized. A few minutes of creative practice will help anyone to understand why we have so many radically different constructs by which to describe nursing—a phenomenon far more complex than our basket.

None of these diverse characterizations of the basket need be inaccurate. The question is not one of right or wrong but of saliency and significance. What is the most useful way to describe the phenomenon? What parts, in what perspective?

In examining a given descriptive theory, many important questions arise such as, was the perception reflective of reality? Did the theorist see the world in the same way as the reader? What constituents did the author accent? What became foreground, what background? Did she select the most important constituents? Did she characterize them in the most salient way?

There are many criteria for determining whether the author succeeded in selecting and characterizing the most important constituents. For now, we will look briefly at one criterion, that of utility, that is, can the theory be used easily? A theory is successful (has selected important constituents) if it is efficient and effective in attaining its socially prescribed goals. In the case of nursing, those goals are outcomes of patient health and comfort that are fully or partly attributable to nursing care. A theory that facilitates the achievement of these nursing goals is successful by the criterion of social utility.

Explanatory Theory

Explanatory theory is the next level in theory development. It attempts to tell how or why the given constituents of a theory relate to and with each other. Explanatory theory may deal with cause and effect, correlations, or the rules that regulate interactions among a theory's constituents. The rules are recognized from study of the patterns established among constituents.

An explanatory theory in its simplest form might assert: When Element A interacts with Element B in Manner Q, then Event M inevitably occurs; when Element A interacts with Element B in Manner R, then Event N inevitably occurs. In other cases, the rules identify probabilities (eg, 90% of the cases) instead of invariant sequences. In nursing there is little that holds true in all cases, except in some cases within the realm of the chemical and biologic.

The test of explanatory theory is whether the prediction holds true in future interactions of the constituents, that is, whether it is *predictive theory*. If, after formulation of the rule, in every new case, Event M follows when Element A interacts with Element B in Manner Q, then the theory has predictive power.

Suppose, for example, that Event N is to be preferred over Event M. Then occurrence of N may be fostered by preventing Manner Q or by facilitating Manner R. When we can manipulate the elements as desired, we have a controlling theory, otherwise called a *situation-producing* theory (Dickoff, James, & Wiedenbach, 1968, p. 420). The explanatory theory itself has not changed. What is altered is the use to which it is put, namely: (1) the time when the theory is applied (predictive theory) or (2) the control possible over elements that act according to the theory's rules (situation-producing theory).

The structure of the theory is identical, be it explanatory, predictive, or situation producing. What differs is our faith in it (test of time) or our ability to control its application in the practice setting according to a set of goals. Some authors assume these are differences in degrees of complexity. This is not the case. One might, for example, have a complex explanation for the rotation of the planets around our sun (explanatory and predictive) without being able to intervene in the planetary system's rotations (situation producing).

EFFECTS OF GOAL DOMINANCE ON THEORY

Most disciplines aim to control their subject matter; they are goal directed. But there are two different ways to gain control over one's subject matter. The chemist, for example, aims to find out what the chemical universe is really like. He does not worry about how he *wishes* the chemical universe acted, he tries to find out how it *does* act. Once he knows how elements react chemically, then he can create conditions to bring about desired chemical reactions.

Similarly, the sociologist studies what makes people act in certain ways. Again, he may wish that people were different, but he seeks to know how they really *are*. Once he knows how people act, he can (if he has the power) create the conditions that bring about desired behaviors and inhibit undesired ones. If, for example, crowded living conditions produce antisocial acts, the enlightened social planner would design buildings for spaciousness. The chemist and the sociologist accept the realities of the worlds of chemistry and human behavior. They take their domains of inquiry as given.

The nurse theorist seldom approaches her domain in this fashion. If a nurse theorist acted like the chemist, she would say, "There's a universe of nursing out there. I'm going to observe it, identify its major elements and events, then find out what rules account for them."

Once the rules that explained the nursing phenomena were found, by following them, she would produce the desired conditions and eliminate the undesired ones. A few nurses advocate this approach to theory building (Quint, 1967; Schlotfeldt, 1971), but they are in the minority. Chapters 3 and 4 offer some illustrations of deriving theory through observation.

Often nurses have an emotional reaction to theory evolved in this manner and say that the theory may describe what some nurses did, but that it does not describe *nursing*. Here is a clue as to how nursing differs from chemistry, sociology, and many other disciplines. The *source* of nursing for many theorists is not the real world of nursing practice; instead, it is a fantasized ideal world of nursing practice as it *would be* if it were done in the best fashion. In this respect, the nurse theorist is unlike the scientist who first seeks to discover the extant state of his subject matter.

This difference in approach is the reason why values creep into almost every discussion of nursing theory. If the source of nursing is in the *ought to be* rather than the *is*, then the values represented in that *ought* are inseparable from nursing. Goals, in turn, are selected on the basis of the given value system. Hence, in nursing, the value system often dictates both the means and the ends to be pursued. For most theorists, nursing is a mentally constructed world rather than the real world of nursing practice. When actual nursing behaviors fall short of the preconceived mental image, the theorist says that it may have been done by nurses, but it was not nursing.

The difference between theory development in nursing and in sociology, then, lies in the *locus* of the subject matter. The nursing discipline usually is located in a mental construct of *ought to be*, whereas sociology is located in the arena of real events and people.

In analyzing any given nursing theory, the reader must ask: Does this theory describe nursing as it *is* or as it *ought to be*? Sometimes an *ought to be* theory is wrongly labeled a situation-producing theory because both are goal dominated. But situation-producing theory also could arise from theory based on *what is*. Most nurse theorists today take their locus for nursing as the *ought*, not the *is*.

THE USE OF COMMONPLACES

Because the location of nursing for most theorists is a mental construct rather than an arena of real events, it is not surprising that there is little agreement on its components. Indeed, there can be as many mental constructs of nursing as there are nurses to imagine them. Even where similar terms are used to describe nursing, their meanings may change from author to author. It is important to differentiate between the terms of a theory and the *commonplaces* into which those terms may be sorted. Commonplaces point to a general location rather than giving specific meanings. For example, a nursing *activity* in one theory may involve hands-on care of the body; in another theory it may represent manipulation of human behavior. A commonplace functions much like labeled desk drawers into which different theorists place different contents.

Content, *methods*, *context*, and *goals* comprise one convenient set of commonplaces that will be used in this book. Alternate lists of commonplaces will be suggested shortly. For each commonplace in a set, one asks: Given this particular theory, what, if anything, fits into this particular sorting bin? The set of containers addressed and omitted, taken together, tells the reader much about the given theory.

Theory analysts create their own sets of commonplaces, and there is no one right set. Analysts concerned with adequacy tend to produce long lists of commonplaces; those concerned with parsimony produce short lists. In their classical work, Dickoff and coworkers (1968) use the following six commonplaces:

> *Agency: Who or what performs the activity?*
> *Patiency: Who or what is the recipient of the activity?*
> *Framework: In what context is the activity performed?*
> *Terminus: What is the end point of the activity?*
> *Procedure: What is the guiding procedure, technique, or protocol of the activity?*
> *Dynamics: What is the energy source for the activity? (p. 423)*

Patiency is a good example from this list. Virtually every nursing theory has some concept of a patient, but the meaning may differ radically from one theory to another. In one, a patient may be a discrete person. Another theory may label a group, community, or organizational entity as patient. Yet another theory may characterize a patient by his entering into a particular type of relationship with a nurse. Another may characterize a patient by specific manifest health needs. One theory may classify the wife of a hospitalized person as *patient* when she learns to balance meals for her diabetic mate. Another theory may claim that patiency resides only in the husband with the health problem.

Duffey and Muhlenkamp (1974) offer a different list of common-places—four questions that form the basis for their evaluation of nursing theories:

> *What is the origin of the problems with which the theory is con-cerned?*
> *What are the methods used?*
> *What is the character of the subject matter dealt with by the theory?*
> *What kind of outcomes of testing propositions generated by this the-ory would you expect to get? (p. 571)*

Roy (1989, pp. 108–113) consciously uses commonplaces in the *construction* of her theory, identifying the following commonplaces:

> *Values*
> *Goals of action*
> *Patiency of the recipient*
> *Source of difficulty*
> *Intervention*

In each case, the selected set of commonplaces tells something about their creator's perspective on nursing. In this sense, the subjec-tive aspect cannot be totally avoided. In addition to analyzing the contents that fall within a set of commonplaces, one can analyze the advantages and limitations inherent in any given set of common-places.

Nurse theorists have always attempted to find general areas of agreement, often in an effort to define a universal theory of nursing. For example, Fawcett (1993, p. 2; 1995, p. 7) identified the components of *person, nursing, health,* and *environment.* Because these terms are commonplaces, and their definitions will vary from one theory to another, they cannot produce a universal theory.

The elements of any theory can be parceled out among any selected set of commonplaces. However, when that task is done, one must also ask what important elements remain. For a complete description of any given theory, one may need to add commonplaces for comprehensiveness. Furthermore, some of the selected commonplaces may not be filled for a given theory.

Mistaken perceptions of universal agreement occur when people agree on the commonplaces to be used rather than on what fills them. Perceived but illusory agreements may arise in superficial reading of theory works when the specific meaning of terms is ignored or misread. Take, for example, the following citation from Newman (1982):

> *The major components of nursing theory are man, environment, and health. As the nurse interacts with man-environment to facilitate health, the nursing process occurs. (p. 87)*

This statement may sound as if Newman were agreeing with Fawcett. However, if one reads further, one sees that Newman is using the terms man, environment, and health in very special ways, that is, in a Rogerian style (Rogers, 1990). The terms cannot be taken to have generic meanings as one might assume from reading the cited sentence out of context. The difference between a commonplace and a theory element is critical: an element is specific to a given theory, a commonplace is not. The reader may wish to see how Flaskerud and Halloran (1980) apply commonplaces to diverse theories.

Words derive their meaning from their function in a given theory and from their relationships to other components of that theory. For example, two nurse theorists may both use the term *adaptation* but mean different things by it. Nor can it be assumed that placing the idea of adaptation in a third theory represents a synthesis of the work of these authors. A term cannot be borrowed from one theory and put into another without changing its meaning. Context contributes to a term's meaning; change the context and you have changed the meaning—even if the word remains.

Another common error in theory development is found at the opposite end of the continuum, that is, groping for certainty by reducing all theory terms to operational definitions. Although the precise, invariant definition of terms is necessary for research, the same tactic may cause premature closure on thoughts and ideas in theory work. For example, if one operationally defines the term *patient* before developing a nursing theory, the direction in which that theory may develop has already been crystallized. In theory development, an initial tolerance for ambiguity is desirable.

Terms may lose the richness of their meaning when operationalized for research. Take the term *adolescence.* It might be operationalized by setting an arbitrary age limit or by validating the occurrence of specified physiologic and sociologic boundary events. But these operationalized definitions are not meant to convey the full significance of the term; they are only meant to enable the researcher to differentiate an adolescent from other people. Although essential for research, operationalized terms can limit conceptualization in theory development.

The reader is asked to suspend the learned desire for concise definition, recognizing that the term *nursing* points only to a general arena of events, and that its specific meaning will be different in every nursing theory.

COMPARING THEORIES

The simplest way to compare and contrast theories is to identify the specific components that make up their respective commonplaces. Take Fawcett's commonplaces of person, nursing, health, and environment for illustration. With this set, one might ask such questions as:

Person
1. Who or what is the "person" in the given theory? Does person refer to the recipient of care alone or does it include the giver of care?
2. Who or what is the patient? Can a group be a patient? Can a society qualify? Can a health care system be the "person" under care?

Nursing
1. Of what do nursing acts consist in the given theory? Thoughts? Activities? Both?
2. Who is able to perform nursing acts? Are there qualifications?

Health
1. What is meant by health in this theory? Is it a continuum from wellness to illness?
2. Is the view of health basically a view of ill health, health deficit, or lack of self-capacity?

3. To what elements of one's existence is health related? Physiologic? Psychological? Spiritual? All aspects of one's being?

Environment
1. What comprises the environment in which nursing occurs? Is it setting bound (eg, an acute care environment)? A long-term care setting?
2. Is the environment interpersonal? Must it involve some form of communication between patient and nurse? Does it involve some contractual sort of relationship?
3. Is the environment mental? Is the environment characterized by a patient's perceived needs or ability to cope?
4. Is the environment physiologically oriented?
5. Is the environment some ecologic notion of the world?

THE NURSING ACT, THE PATIENT, THE INTERACTION

Theories also differ as to which commonplaces are stressed. Most nursing theories place their basic principles in one of three loci:

1. The nursing act
2. The patient
3. The relationship between patient and nursing act (the interaction itself)

In the first instance, the unstated assumption is that by knowing what the nurse does (or should do) one comes to understand nursing. The second focus implies that if we really understand the patient, then knowledge of nursing acts logically follows. The third stance does not place the essence of nursing in the acts or conditions of any human agent but in the particular character of the interchange between patient and nurse.

Major trends in nursing theory can be attributed to these three alternative emphases. For example, the focus on nurses and what they do is illustrated by the nursing process. The American Nurses Association's (ANA) advocacy of the nursing process (it appears in almost all ANA standards of practice) has done much to make the nursing act dominant.

In contrast, a focus on the patient is evident in nursing curricula structured around body systems. Here, if one knows the patient, namely his body systems, the correct nursing acts logically will follow. Curricula based on patient problems (pain, anxiety, immobility) also select the patient as the focus. Holistic theories typically make the patient their focus although they see the patient in a different light than the older body systems orientation.

Curricula and practice based on nursing diagnoses often mix these two elements in disorderly array. For example, a nursing diagnosis of respiratory distress is centered in the patient, whereas a diagnosis of negative appraisal by others (Carpenito, 1984, p. 74) may be more the nurse's problem. Later editions (eg, Carpenito, 1997) are less likely to make this type of error.

A focus on the interaction itself is evident in the works of King and Watson. King's (1981, pp. 60–62) approach is existential, confirming that interaction occurs between patient and nurse, with transaction (agreement between patient and nurse on a goal with movement toward achievement of the goal) as the culminating act. Watson's (1988, p. 57) notion of caring creates a different sort of interactions theory. Her transaction simultaneously contributes to the patient's and nurse's development of spiritual essence, self-knowledge, and self-healing. Existential theories of nursing often focus on the "I–Thou" type of interaction.

DRAWING BOUNDARIES AROUND THE PROFESSION

Although it is necessary to tolerate ambiguity, it is equally important that any specific nursing theory—directly or by implication—differentiate nursing from other disciplines and activities. Many so-called theories of nursing fail in this aspect, creating a schema that could apply equally well to medicine, physical therapy, social work, or general caretaking. These theories have failed to settle the boundary issue.

The so-called nursing process can be criticized for this fault. The electrical engineer, the architect, the nuclear scientist, as well as the school counselor, all assess, diagnose, plan, intervene, and evaluate. One could easily talk about the architectural process or the counseling process. Only when this common process is tied to specific content (additional theory elements) can one say the boundary has been drawn successfully around a discipline.

When authors fail to differentiate nursing, the error usually is found in one of two directions: either the theory is equally applicable to (1) medicine and other health professions or (2) to nonprofessional activities such as mothering, caring, and nurturing.

Theories based on stress–adaptation models often fail to differentiate nursing from other health professions. A good test for this error is to substitute the word *medicine* (or social work) for the word *nursing* every time it appears in a theory. If the work remains cogent and applicable in the substituted discipline, then the theory has failed to distinguish nursing from other health professions.

A theory that defines nursing primarily by its intent or effect, without reference to the skills unique to nursing, may fail in the opposite direction, not differentiating nursing from the general caring acts of humans for one another. Some theories based on caring models fall into this error. Try substituting the term *mother* or *caring human being* for *nurse* in these theories to test for the flaw.

THE BASIS FOR NURSING

A theory can successfully differentiate nursing from other disciplines and human activities on several bases. Is nursing unique because it has a separate body of knowledge? Because it uses shared knowledge in a distinct manner? Because it comes into being in a unique set of circumstances? Or because it has discrete goals?

The first interpretation differentiates nursing in terms of its substantive *content*, the second in terms of its method and practices, (ie, *processes*), the third in terms of the *context* in which it occurs, and the last in terms of its *goals*. Each interpretation presents its own difficulties.

Where nursing's uniqueness lies in knowledge (content) rather than in action, the knowledge must be separate and unlike that taught to other health disciplines. The problem here is one of finding content so unique that no other discipline lays claim to it. Rogers (1990, p. 6), for example, asserts that nursing's unique subject matter is the science of unitary human beings, man in his totality rather than seen in component parts.

When a nursing theory develops a truly unique body of knowledge, it has the problem of communicating its meaning to other health disciplines. When nursing's subject matter is radically different, its distinct language presents interface problems in situations where different professions work closely together. This does not mean that nursing cannot develop separate theories; it simply means that one considers what is to be gained and what lost in this tactic. In adopting a theory that has a radically different conceptualization of man (or his care) than the theories used by other health workers in the care environment, one runs the danger of increasing problems in interprofessional communication.

When a radically divergent nursing theory is selected, nursing has the task of helping others understand its unique language or translating its programs into language that others can understand. Where communication bridges are not devised, cooperative work is difficult. Many theorists argue, however, that creating separate content for nursing is worth the price of problematic communications because it establishes a clear and separate identity for nursing.

When nursing's uniqueness lies in the *use* of knowledge rather than in the knowledge itself, then one must show how nursing bridges from shared content to unique action. One must identify which acts are particularized to nursing and why. What groups share the content that each applies differently? Medicine? Social work? How is the application different?

Some theories that find nursing's boundaries in its *use* of knowledge see it as a generalist practice arising from the blending of content from other disciplines. With this interpretation, one must tell how to synthesize content from various disciplines (eg, medicine, anatomy, psychology, and sociology) when the nurse is not an expert in any of them. Here the nurse theorist faces the awesome task of explaining how one derives a generalist's discipline from little-studied specialty fields.

Perhaps the most difficult boundary to understand is where the *circumstance* (or context) differentiates nursing from other disciplines. In written theories, a context often is assumed rather than stated. Some theorists, for example, have an underlying image of nursing as constituted by all those acts between nurse and patient in an acute care hospital setting. In this example, an act becomes nursing, not because of its content or method, but because it occurs in a particular setting where a nurse and patient are brought together.

Consider a different context. Suppose a nurse is talking to a neighbor who asks about a health-related problem. When does *nursing*, as opposed to casual conversation, begin? Or does it? What situational variants define the context as a nursing situation?

Nor is theory easier if the difference is to be made on the basis of *goals*. Here a unique complexity arises because nursing contributes toward achievement of medical as well as nursing goals. When nurses perform an act aimed toward medical goals, are they nursing? If not, what are they doing? The answer to this question is critical in a program that prepares advanced nurse practitioners for primary care delivery.

INTERPRETING NURSING THEORIES

Theorists do not make the job of identifying commonplaces easy. Seldom will a theorist state, in so many words, that the image of patient is a hospitalized individual under medical care. Yet if every reference to patient is given from this perspective, and nursing, as described, takes place only when a person is in this state, then the reader can infer that this description of patient (patiency) fits.

One cannot take a theorist too literally. For example, a theorist may start out with a definition of patient as an individual, group of persons, or community. But if all further discussion only addresses the patient as an individual, the theorist's original definition was simply a slogan. The real definition is *that characterization intrinsic to the given theory*.

Many theorists fall into the trap of using slogans, particularly those in vogue at the time their material was written. One sees theorists who claim that the patient is a full-fledged participant in determining his plan of nursing care, yet fail to apply the concept in the theory that follows. *Sloganism* is a claim put forth but not substantiated in the theory elaboration. The reader may be suspicious of any of the following claims until substantiated:

1. The nurse is a problem solver.
2. The patient participates in his care determination.
3. Health is a state of total well-being.
4. The nurse uses the nursing process.
5. The theory uses a systems approach to nursing.
6. Caring is the basis of all nursing actions.
7. The presented theory is holistic.

NURSING THEORY AND CRITICAL THINKING

The methods of theory inquiry given here are highly analytical. Hence, the study of nursing theory is closely allied with the development of critical thinking skills. Indeed, the intellectual tools needed to understand theory are exactly those abilities required in clinical critical thinking. I disapprove of the National League for Nursing engendered criterion of "critical thinking" because all of nursing should require critical thinking. It should not be chopped off and offered like a block on a separate plate. For example, clinical critical thinking requires the three skills of recognizing, interpreting, and adapting. An instance of each of these skills will be examined here: red flagging, labeling, and responding.

Red Flagging

Red flagging means recognizing that a problem situation exists. In a negative example, I observed a nurse complete a nursing history for a patient, during which she asked if the patient had any chronic health problems. The patient responded negatively. Two questions later she asked if he were routinely taking any medications. The patient responded that he took Aldactazide daily. The nurse wrote in this fact and continued down the form. No red flag was raised in her mind when a patient who claimed *no* chronic health problem admitted to taking a drug daily. This failure of critical thinking cannot be accounted for simply as a lack of knowledge concerning the drug. Whether or not she knew the drug, she should have recognized the inconsistency in the patient's two responses.

Labeling

Labeling allows a nurse to interpret a concrete situation by virtue of previously acquired concepts. Acquisition of the pertinent concept(s) alone does not ensure application in the clinical setting. For example, the nurse may have a general conception of *denial*, but something in the patient's behavior must trigger the nurse's judgment that denial exists. Interpreting is complex in that understanding of a concept is a precondition, but identification of the concept in its unique instantiation is required.

Critical thinking involves recognizing diverse and varying instances of the concept. Psychic states such as denial, anxiety, and euphoria take different forms in different patients. Similarly, physiologic states vary in symptomatology among patients. One cannot be assumed to have grasped a concept through identifying a single, or even several, instantiations.

Responding

Responding involves an appropriate response to a problem. As an illustration, I once observed a nursing staff caring for a patient on absolute voice rest. Each nurse entered the room, reminded the patient of the need for voice rest, then posed questions requiring verbal responses. The nurses' own behaviors elicited the forbidden response. Only one nurse developed a successful response: whispering to the patient. The deviation in her own vocal behavior was a successful reminder to the patient.

Red flagging, labeling, and responding form a bridge between cognitive content (abstract and general) and extant instantiations of that content (concrete and specific). Aspects such as this are the essence of critical thinking. Although no course substitutes for clinical learning, a well taught course of nursing theory teaches students the habit of making such discriminations. In a theory course taught as an analytical task, students inevitably report that their reading habits change. They look at things differently in other courses and in their private and professional lives as well. They start asking of what they read: Does it make sense? Do I believe the arguments? What is missing? This skill carries well past reading into practice.

What is missing from this patient's picture? Why isn't that patient responding to my intervention?

SUMMARY

Structural devices help the reader to understand a theory and to compare theories in a systematic fashion. These devices include determining whether the theory is descriptive or explanatory—as well as its level of development. The boundaries drawn around nursing determine how it is different from other activities. Commonplaces addressed or omitted and the meanings given to each component slotted into a commonplace describe the theory. Among commonplace sets, one includes the elements of content, process, context, and goal. Learning to interpret theory is the key; a theory must be understood, not merely memorized like a procedure. Analytical tools are the means for enhancing one's understanding of theories.

PRACTICE EXERCISE

Analyze one or more theoretical statements of limited size, perhaps 4 to 6 pages. Carefully read and reread the given theory piece, asking the following questions or completing the identified tasks.

1. *Identify the major elements of the theory.*
   Which commonplace elements are present? Which are missing? What item fills each commonplace? Determine each of the stated or implied commonplaces: content, process, context, and goal.
2. *Determine whether the theory is descriptive or explanatory.*
   Does the theory simply tell what exists? Does the theory tell why and how?
3. *Determine if the theory describes nursing as it is or as it should be.*
   Does the theory describe what nurses do or what nurses ought to do?
4. *Tell how nursing in this theory differs from other domains.*
   On what basis is it bounded? Does the theory distinguish nursing from medicine or other health fields? Does it distinguish nursing from other aspects of life unrelated to health (eg, normal social interaction)? Does nursing differ from simple caring acts?
5. *Tell whether the crux of nursing rests in the content of nursing knowledge, in the methods of performing nursing acts, in the nursing context, or in its goals.*

6. *Identify whether the main locus of the theory is in the patient, the nursing act, or the nurse–patient relationship.*
   Do the terms used by the author focus on the patient (or elements of his being), the nurse (or her acts), or on the relationship between patient and nurse?
7. *Identify slogans used by the author.*
   Did the theorist give any definitions inconsistent with the theory? Were any claims asserted and then dropped from subsequent discussion?

REFERENCES

Carpenito, L. J. (1984). *Handbook of nursing diagnosis*. Philadelphia: Lippincott.

Carpenito, L. J. (1997). *Handbook of nursing diagnosis* (7th ed). Philadelphia: Lippincott-Raven.

Dickoff, J., James, P., & Wiedenbach, E. (1968, September/October). Theory in a practice discipline: Part I. Practice oriented theory. *Nursing Research, 5*, 415–435.

Duffey, M., & Muhlenkamp, A. F. (1974, September). A framework for theory analysis. *Nursing Outlook, 9*, 571–574.

Fawcett, J. (1993). *Analysis and evaluation of nursing theories*. Philadelphia: Davis.

Fawcett, J. (1995). *Analysis and evaluation of conceptual models of nursing*. Philadelphia: Davis.

Flaskerud, J. H., & Halloran, E. J. (1980, October). Areas of agreement in nursing theory development. *Advances in Nursing Science, 1*, 1–7.

King, I. (1981). *A theory for nursing: Systems, concepts, process*. New York: Wiley.

Levine, M. E. (1971, June). Holistic nursing. *Nursing Clinics of North America, 2*, 253–264.

Newman, M. A. (1982, October). What differentiates clinical research? *Image, 3*, 86–88.

Quint, J. C. (1967, Spring). The case for theories generated from empirical data. *Nursing Research, 2*, 109–114.

Rogers, M. E. (1990). Nursing: Science of unitary, irreducible, human beings: Update 1990. In E. A. M. Barrett (Ed.), *Visions of Roger's science-based nursing* (pp. 5–11). New York: National League for Nursing.

Roy, C. (1989). The Roy adaptation model. In J. Riehl-Sisca (Ed.), *Conceptual models for nursing practice* (3rd ed., pp. 105–114). New York: Appleton-Century-Crofts.

Schlotfeldt, R. M. (1971, March/April). The significance of empirical research for nursing. *Nursing Research, 2*, 140–142.

Visintainer, M. A. (1986, Summer). The nature of knowledge and theory in nursing. *Image, 2*, 32–38.

Watson, J. (1988). *Nursing: Human science and human care: A theory of nursing*. New York: National League for Nursing.

2 *Structure Underlying Theory*

COMPREHENSIVE THEORY ELEMENTS

Chapter 1 mentioned the use of commonplaces, context, content, process, and goal, as tools for analyzing works of nursing theory. This chapter examines these notions in greater detail. A complete theory of nursing identifies all four elements: context, content, process, and goal. These elements are envisioned as a magic carpet on which a design has been embossed. The original unadorned rug may be equated with the context, that is, the background on which other elements play. The threads of the embossed design are envisioned to cross-hatch so that those running horizontally represent content, whereas those running vertically are equated with process. Content and process interact on the background, that is, the context. The fourth element, goal, is the direction in which the magic carpet is flying.

Context is the *environment* in which nursing acts occur. It tells the nature of the world of nursing and, in most cases, this involves describing the salient characteristics of the patient's surroundings. For example, Roy (1980, 1989) sees a world characterized by the dominance of stimulus—response reactions. In this sort of world, the nurse manipulates stimuli; the patient responds.

Content is the *subject matter* of a theory; it is comprised of the stable elements that are acted on or that do the acting. For example, Levine (1967, 1989) offers energy, structure, personal integrity, and social integrity as her content components.

Process is the *method* by which the theory works. It is the dynamic element, usually found in the nursing acts or thoughts. It can usually be found in the form of a verb. Process happens when the nurse acts on, with, or through the content pieces of the theory. Often the patient and nurse have complementary processes: Levine's nurse conserves, her patient adapts; Roy's nurse manipulates stimuli; her patient responds. Sometimes patient and nurse share the same process: King's (1981) nurse and patient act, react, and (together) transact; Orem's (1985) patient and nurse both deliver self-care.

The *goal* is the intended *aim* of the theory, what the nurse hopes to achieve. Obviously, the aim can be different from the actual outcome, but the goal states the intended end of the nursing endeavor. In an era when outcomes management is the rule, we see many goal statements, for example, in patient standards, in case maps, and in accreditation standards. Similarly, a complete theory identifies the goal so one can know if the theory has achieved its intended result.

CONTEXT

What counts as significant context differs from theory to theory. It may be the nature of the planet itself (eg, in ecofeminism), it may be the nature of the patient's immediate environment (eg, the acute care hospital world), or it may be the nature of human beings themselves (as in Roy's stimulus–response connotation). Whatever context is important to a theory, it describes the nature of the background in which nursing occurs.

Johnson (1980) has a context whereby the nurse works in a world of behavior. The patient exhibits behaviors; the nurse manipulates his drives and needs to create desired changes in behavior. This does not mean that the entire universe is made up only of behavior, but for Johnson behavior is the domain in which nursing occurs. In contrast, Rubin (1968) has a context described as the eternally changing present. The idea of the moment and the fluidity of circumstances characterize the environment for her. For Leininger (1991), the patient's culture is the important context.

Some theorists spell out context better than others. Watson (1988) specifically defines the "human science" context in which her theory is located:

- *A philosophy of human freedom, choice, and responsibility*
- *A biology and psychology of holism (nonreducible persons interconnected with others and nature)*
- *An epistemology that allows not only for empirics, but for advancement of esthetics, ethical values, intuition, and process discovery*

- *An ontology of time and space*
- *A context of interhuman events, processes, and relationships*
- *A scientific world view that is open (p. 16)*

After one reads such a list, it is easy to imagine what sort of nursing would fit—or would not fit—in such a world.

Nor is context always captured in a single notion or a finite set of principles like Watson's. Hall's (1966) context is chronic illness. It is also accurate to say that her context is one of existential crisis in which man's capacity for radical, free choice characterizes the environment. Both of these aspects would reflect context because her nurse helps the rehabilitation patient (who has chronic, incurable conditions) strive to reach an existential goal of mental and psychological self-mastery.

Chopoorian (1986) notes that there are many significant environments: (1) the social, political, and economic structures; (2) human or social relations; and (3) everyday life. A theory of nursing can present many different, yet not inconsistent, environments. Context is the category that extracts the most important environments, the ones that are essential to understanding the theory.

In many nursing theories the context is unstated and must be inferred from the general discussion. For example, one might find a theory in which the context is the acute care hospital dealing with ill patients. In a better detailed theory, one might find a context of health deficit or one in which homeostasis is the key to the patient's world. These examples, both illness based, might be contrasted with a theory in which even the well need nursing.

Donovan (1970) is one of the rare theorists who carefully identifies context, classifying sources of nursing by contextual factors: (1) derived—through the medical plan, (2) fluctuating—relinquished from others (eg, the pharmacist), (3) coordinative—elements resulting from the holding position of the nurse in relation to the patient, and (4) independent—those elements that are distinctly nursing.

Finer (1952, pp. 88, 90) gives a different description of context, noting that nursing occurs in an environment characterized by continuousness, diversity of needs, contingency, and high emotionality. By continuous, he means the nurse's 24-hour, uninterrupted vigilance over the patient. By diversity of needs, he means the need to individualize patient care planning. Contingency refers to the ever-changing nature of the patient's needs and the fact that nursing acts must be adjusted on an ongoing basis. High emotionality refers to the life and death and stress-filled situations faced by patients, requiring compassion and understanding on the part of the nurse.

More recently, Leininger (1991, p. 43), in her ethnonursing model, makes a context of cultural and social structures: technological factors, religious and philosophical factors, kinship and social factors, cultural values and lifeways, political and legal factors, economic factors, and educational factors.

Differences in context among theorists illustrate a shift over time in the nursing viewpoint. Older theories, such as those of Donovan and Finer, tended to portray the image of an acute care hospital. Newer theories (eg, Leininger or Chopoorian) tend to see nursing in more diverse or multiple contexts. In a time when much nursing care is shifting from the acute care setting to home and community, this shift in theory context is to be expected.

CONTENT

Content is used here to identify the relatively stable theory elements that are the subject matter of a nursing theory. Often the subject elements are the categories through which nursing acts are accomplished. For Johnson (1980), content consists of the categories of patient behavior: elimination behavior, sexual behavior, and so forth. For Roy (1980), content includes the four adaptation modes of man: physiologic needs, self-concept, role function, and interdependence relations. For Neuman (1980), content includes but is not limited to energy resources, stressors, and lines of resistance.

Not all theorists limit their basic content to aspects of the patient. For King (1981), one set of content items would be personal systems, interpersonal relationships, and social systems. Roger's (1970) components are even broader, consisting of man (human field), environmental field, space, time, and innovation.

Content intersects with both process and context to make a complete theory. The interaction with process may be illustrated in the theories built around the so-called nursing process. In this theory (there are many variations on the theme), the nursing process (assess, diagnose, plan, intervene, evaluate) is linked to a taxonomy of nursing diagnoses. These diagnoses, the most common arising from the work of the North American Nursing Diagnosis Association (1996), represent the content part of the theory.

For an excellent example of content interacting with context, see Strauss, Fagerhaugh, and Glaser (1974). These authors, in a narrow range theory, consider how content (pain) is affected by context (the "normal" pain trajectories for the given work areas). They find that different areas in the same institution (altered contexts) deal with pain in radically different ways.

Content items, then, are the main theory building blocks that give a theory form without being the moving forces. The moving forces constitute the processes.

PROCESS

Processes may be stated as nouns or verbs, but in either case, they represent the movement, the dynamic part of the theory. The processes (or process) of a theory refer to those activities (intellectual, affective, or behavioral) on the part of the agent (nurse or patient) that are required to implement the theory. For Hall (1966), process elements include mirroring, nurturing, and comforting on the part of the nurse and self-mastery on the part of the patient. For Levine (1971), nurses conserve; patients adapt, but the specifics are not well developed directives. For example, she says:

> *The integrated response of the individual to any stimulus results in a realignment of his very substance, and in a sense this creates a message which others may learn to understand. Each message, in turn, is the result of observation, selection of relevant data, and assessment of the priorities demanded by such knowledge. (Levine, 1967, p. 46)*

This statement is Levine's only indication of how the conservation process proceeds. This format, incidentally, is typical of a problematic approach because different problems require different methods.

For Newman (1979), the nurse's process is to help the patient expand his consciousness by ". . . assist(ing) people to utilize the power that is within them as they evolve toward higher levels of consciousness" (pp. 66–67). Her process (1994) is that of helping the patient *repattern* those patterns and structures (traits, behaviors, choices) that characterize him, in other words, realigning his very being.

Almost invariably, the process items of a theory act on or through the content items of the theory. For example, in Orem (1985, p. 92), self-care (an action, ie, a process) is applied in the content domains of: (1) air, water, and food; (2) excrements; (3) rest and activity; and so forth. Roy (1980, p. 182), in contrast, operates on a microlevel. Her nurse manipulates stimulus–response (process) in the content domains of: (1) physiologic needs, (2) self-concept needs, (3) role function, and (4) interdependence.

For some theorists process is reduced to a single activity, for example, problem-solving. For others, numerous processes are involved. Orem (1985, p. 92) illustrates both points because her theory is based on a major process, self-care. Yet the specific forms for self care differ with each content item. For example, she speaks of maintenance (process) of sufficient intake of air, water, food (content), or provision of care (process) associated with elimination processes and excrements (content).

In another section of the book, Orem (1985) classifies these processes in a different manner, according to the method of giving assistance:

1. *Acting for or doing for another*
2. *Guiding another*
3. *Supporting another (physically or psychologically)*
4. *Providing an environment that promotes personal development in relation to becoming able to meet present or future demands for action*
5. *Teaching another (p. 138)*

Two common process theory threads in nursing are the nursing process and problem-solving. Both are discussed in later chapters. Either of these processes may be combined with differing contents, contrasting goals, and varying contexts. The processes will be somewhat changed according to the context, goal, and content with which they are combined.

Other processes are certainly possible in nursing; they are just not as common. It is surprising, for example, that nursing has not created a popular theory based on the method of differential diagnosis as has been done in medicine. Some developing theories of nurse practitioner action are looking at this approach, however. Orem's original theory comes closest to this operational pattern, that is, making either/or choices at each step.

In some theories, the dialectic process of *synthesis* is the method of choice. The term synthesis often is used in nursing literature, but the process itself is seldom used in practice. Sometimes nurses claim to be synthesizing when they are actually accumulating (adding) data or activities. Synergism is different from a mere adding together of parts. Brodt (1980) is one theorist who uses the notion of synthesis or synergism accurately. However, she uses it in relation to goal achievement rather than in relation to a nursing process. She says:

> *The synergistic theory of nursing postulates that nursing practice consists of six dimensions of practice, which when delivered to the client simultaneously and interrelatedly provide the optimum level of care and the most positive outcome for the client. (p. 85)*
>
> *As a corollary, the effect of each dimension of nursing practice enhances the other dimensions when presented simultaneously and interrelatedly. The effect is similar to the synergistic action of two drugs on the human body, in which the combined action is different from the effect*

of either drug taken independently. In the combined administration of the nursing dimensions, the whole also is greater than the sum of its parts. (p. 87)

The dimensions of Brodt's theory include preservation of body defenses, prevention of complications, maintenance or reestablishment of the client with the outside world, detection of changes in the body's regulatory system, implementation of the physician's prescribed therapy, and provision of comfort and safety. Notice that each item contains both content and process. This format was common in early theory works where each process was identified with a specific content. Thus we see that, for Brodt, preservation (process) relates to body defenses (content); prevention (process) relates to complication (content), and so forth. Compare this to the newer format in which one process, for example, conservation, is applied to numerous categorical (not ad hoc) content items.

Although Brodt describes synthesis as a *result*, Newman (1979) describes it as a dialectic *process*:

A holistic approach is not to be confused with, or construed to mean, a multivariate approach. It is not the summing up of many factors (psychological, social, physiological, and so on) to make a whole. It is the identification of patterns which are reflective of the whole. (p. 70)

Not surprisingly, Newman claims that phenomenology offers nurses the opportunity to observe these patterns of the whole.

As with Newman, the process in a given theory not only tells how the nurse performs (intellectually and behaviorally), but also indicates appropriate methods of research and teaching behavior. For the same theory, processes in these domains should be consonant if not identical.

Often the processes of a theory are termed its syntactical structures. As Ziman (1968) says:

To understand the nature of Science, we must look at the way in which scientists behave toward one another, how they are organized and how information passes between them. The young scientist does not study formal logic, but he learns by imitation and experience a number of conventions that embody strong social relationships. (p. 10)

GOAL

The goal element in nursing theory is the intended outcome of the nursing effort. For Roy (1980), the intent is to relieve the patient of his focus on the present stimuli (the stimuli related to his pain or associated with his illness) and free his attention for other stimuli. More simply put, Roy (1989) says the goal is adaptation in all four of her content modes. For Hall (1966), the goal is the patient's self-mastery despite his bodily limitations. In this example, the process of self-mastery (verb) can lead to the goal of self-mastery (noun).

Some of the newer holistic nursing theories have goals that are spiritual in nature. Watson (1988) wants the patient to achieve harmony of body, mind, and spirit, and Newman (1994) sees the goal as the patient's continuous evolution to higher levels of consciousness.

INTERPLAY

Few theories are complete in their descriptions of context, content, process, and goal. Theorists often focus on one or two of these structural constituents, giving minimal attention to the remaining ones. For example, Donovan and Finer stress context. Johnson (1980) stresses content (eg, behavioral systems). On the other hand, her attention to process is less well formulated:

> Nursing is thus seen as an external regulatory force which acts to preserve the organization and integration of the patient's behavior at an optimal level under those conditions in which the behavior constitutes a threat to physical or social health, or in which illness is found. This force operates through the imposition of external regulatory or control mechanisms, through attempts to change structural units in desirable directions, or through the fulfillment of the functional requirements of the subsystems. (p. 214)

In contrast to Johnson's brief clarification of her processes, Peplau is highly process oriented. For example, in a psychiatric nursing context, she spells out the unique processes for managing frustration, anxiety, and other phenomena. Given the content of patient anxiety, she identifies process steps to accompany every aspect of the patient experience (Peplau, 1989, pp. 24–25). For example, when the patient voices an upsetting expectation, the nurse connects the anxiety and the expectation (process). When the patient subsequently experiences discomfort and internal tension, the nurse names the experience as anxiety. Peplau continues this step-by-step attention to process throughout the whole anxiety experience, with nursing process tied to each step of the patient's experience. We really have two processes at work in Peplau's discussion, the patient's experiential process and the nurse's response process. One of the charms of Peplau for many nurses is that her work gives these concrete steps to be taken. Others, however, are frustrated by the number of components that thereby accrue in her work.

Some theorists compose one theory and stick by it; others grow and let their theory develop. For example, the early work by Levine is light on process. In contrast, Levine's later work (1973, pp. 7–9) details the patient's process (maintaining a homeostatic balance between an upper and lower normal limit) and the nurse's intervention (exercising control over negative feedback in regulatory systems).

Levine addresses two different contexts in her early theory, with the explanation of structural and energy conservation built on a context of disease, that is, the patient's condition was the basis. In contrast, her explanation of personal and social integrity was built on the context of the hospital (the negative aspects of being in an institutional setting). This reflects the tension many nurse theorists develop in trying to deal with normative physiologic data and unique personal, humanistic information in the same theory.

In her later work, Levine (1989) focuses much more on environment, noting that there are three environments: the environment of living tissues (eg, radiation, microorganisms), the sensate environment (eg, taste, touch), and the environment of perception (eg, thinking, symbols, awareness of the past). Concerning man as patient, she says:

> The environment is often seen as a passive backdrop against which the individual "acts out" life experiences. But an individual cannot be understood outside of the context of his or her predicament of time and place. Only then are the "open and fluid" boundaries established. (p. 326)

Theories can be uneven regarding the attention given to context, content, process, and goals. Some theorists focus on one or two elements to the exclusion of others. Often the reader will be able to infer the other items, even though they are not well developed. At times, however, it will be impossible to determine the nature of the missing elements. It may appear that the same term fills two commonplaces. For example, a theory might have adaptation as a process (really the verb, adapt) and adaptation (the noun) as the goal.

SUMMARY

If a theory is complete it includes clear definitions or descriptions of context, content, process, and goal. It also provides the reader with an understanding of how these components interrelate. As commonplaces, context, content, process, and goal provide a matrix, an organizing framework through which a theory can be understood or compared to other theories. Table 2–1 gives a sample of how such elements might look for a few theorists. (Some degree of accuracy and complexity has been sacrificed in the table to achieve the brief comparisons.)

Table 2–1. *Comparison of Theories*

Theorist	Content	Process	Context	Goal
Roy	Physiologic needs, self-concept needs, role function, interdependence	Nurse manipulates stimuli; patient responds to stimuli	Stimulus–response theory of human adjustment	Adjusted in all four modes
King	Personal systems, interpersonal relationships, social systems	Patient and nurse: perception, judgment, action, reaction, transaction	Interpersonal systems	Agreement on a goal between nurse and patient
Orem	Self-care universals or health deviation self-care needs	Self-care by nurse, then by patient	Deficit in ability to satisfy required self-care needs	Return of self-care to the patient
Levine (early)	Structural integrity, energy, personal integrity, social integrity	Conserving by nurse; adapting by patient	Problem-solving environment	Adaptation, problem resolution
Johnson	Behavior systems, eg, eliminative behavior, aggressive behavior, etc.	Nurse manipulates behavioral responses intervening through goals, drives, needs	World of human behavior	Socially approved behavior
Rogers	Human field, environmental field, energy field, pattern, multidimensionality	Resonancy, helicy, integrality	World of continuously evolving man	Continuous innovative evolution of man and environment

REFERENCES

Brodt, D. E. (1980). A re-examination of the synergistic theory of nursing. *Nursing Forum, 1,* 85–93.

Chopoorian, T. J. (1986). Reconceptualizing the environment. In P. Moccia (Ed.), *New approaches to theory development* (pp. 39–54). New York: National League for Nursing Press.

Donovan, H. M. (1970, October). Toward a definition of nursing. *Supervisor Nurse, 5,* 12–15.

Finer, H. (1952). *Administration and the nursing services.* New York: Macmillan.

Hall, L. E. (1966). Another view of nursing care and quality. In K. M. Straub & K. S. Parker (Eds.), *Continuity of patient care: The role of nursing* (pp. 47–60). Washington, DC: Catholic University Press of America.

Johnson, D. E. (1980). Behavioral system model for nursing. In J. P. Riehl & C. Roy (Eds.), *Conceptual models for nursing practice* (2nd ed., pp. 207–216). New York: Appleton-Century-Crofts.

King, I. (1981). *A theory for nursing: Systems, concepts, process,* New York: Wiley.

Leininger, M. M. (1991). The theory of culture care diversity and universality. In M. M. Leininger (Ed.), *Culture care diversity & universality: A theory of nursing* (pp. 5–68). New York: National League for Nursing.

Levine, M. E. (1967). The four conservation principles of nursing. *Nursing Forum, 1,* 45–59.

Levine, M. E. (1971, June). Holistic nursing. *Nursing Clinics of North America, 2,* 253–264.

Levine, M. E. (1973). *Introduction to clinical nursing* (2nd ed.). Philadelphia: Davis.

Levine, M. E. (1989). The conservation principles of nursing: Twenty years later. In J. Riehl-Sisca (Ed.), *Conceptual models for nursing practice* (3rd ed., pp. 325–337). Norwalk, CT: Appleton & Lange.

Neuman, B. (1980). The Betty Neuman health-care systems model: A total person approach to patient problems. In J. P. Riehl & C. Roy (Eds.), *Conceptual models for nursing practice* (2nd ed., pp. 119–134). New York: Appleton-Century-Crofts.

Newman, M. A. (1979). *Theory development in nursing.* Philadelphia: Davis.

Newman, M. A. (1994). *Health as expanding consciousness.* New York: National League for Nursing Press.

North American Nursing Diagnosis Association (NANDA). (1996). *Nursing diagnoses: Definitions and classification 1997–1998.* Philadelphia: Author.

Orem, D. E. (1985). *Nursing: Concepts of practice* (3rd ed.). New York: McGraw-Hill.

Peplau, H. E. (1989). Theory: The professional dimension. In A. W. O'Toole & S. R. Welt (Eds.), *Interpersonal theory in nursing practice: Selected works of Hildegard E. Peplau.* New York: Springer.

Rogers, M. E. (1970). *An introduction to the theoretical basis of nursing.* Philadelphia: Davis.

Roy, C. (1980). The Roy adaptation model. In J. P. Riehl & C. Roy (Eds.), *Conceptual models for nursing practice* (2nd ed., pp. 183–187). New York: Appleton-Century-Crofts.

Roy, C. (1989). The Roy adaptation model. In J. Riehl-Sisca (Ed.), *Conceptual models for nursing practice* (3rd ed., pp. 105–114). Norwalk, CT: Appleton & Lange.

Rubin, R. (1968, May/June). A theory of clinical nursing. *Nursing Research*, *3*, 210–212.

Strauss, A., Fagerhaugh, S. Y., & Glaser, B. (1974, September). Pain: An organizational-work-interactional perspective. *Nursing Outlook*, *9*, 560–566.

Watson, J. (1988). *Nursing: Human science and human care: A theory of nursing.* New York: National League for Nursing.

Ziman, J. (1968). *Public knowledge: The social dimension of science,* London: Cambridge University Press.

3 The Normative Theory of Nursing

Before nursing leaders ever thought about nursing theory, nurses and nurse educators still managed to work and teach effectively. Indeed, generations of nurses educated without reference to nursing theory perceived no shortcomings in their preparation. Despite the absence of a nursing theory, there was general consensus on what should be included in nursing education and what a nurse should and should not do in practice.

This chapter explores these shared expectations from the perspective of theory development. What is the unexplicated but shared theory of nursing that governs general practice? What are the generally accepted tenets around which nursing education and practice are structured?

It may be of value for the reader to brainstorm (as an individual or in a group) on these questions before reading further. Any nurse can easily come up with a list of precepts and rules that apply in nursing practice. The reader may be interested to see if his or her list is similar to that given in this chapter (derived from numerous classes of graduate students).

The objective of this exercise is to make the reader cognizant of the unstated expectations that influence the way in which nurses go about their work. These are the expectations that, if unmet, make a peer group question a nurse's performance. We will call these expectations *premises* of nursing practice because they underlie the way nurses practice. They constitute an operative theory of nursing, albeit uncodified.

The following values, beliefs, and operating rules are usually identified when a group of nurses examine the assumed bases of nursing action. The first set concerns the nurse's beliefs about the patient:

- Pain is bad (except when needed for diagnosis); relief is to be desired.
- Anxiety is bad; a relaxed state of mind is to be preferred.
- Knowledge of one's condition and its management is to be preferred over ignorance.
- In most cases, knowledge of one's prognosis is to be preferred over ignorance.
- Independence is to be preferred over dependence.

These patient-based premises underlie the actions and approaches taken by most nurses. They could be restated as nursing principles for action, for example, the nurse should relieve anxiety, the nurse should alleviate pain.

The next group of factors relate to how nurses present themselves or how they act. They:

- Never reveal repugnance for sights or smells. They mask any revulsion caused by putrefaction, vomitus, body excreta, or human disfigurement.
- Never display unwillingness to serve patients. They present themselves as pleased to render any legitimate service of whatever nature.
- Never reveal their own anxieties and fears, but present a facade of professional control in all situations.
- Relieve the patient's embarrassment by dealing matter of factly with levels of intimacy that are unusual in other settings; for example, assuring patients that exposed bodies are routine for nurses and that they should not be embarrassed during intimate care procedures.
- Provide reassurance as a basic mode of interacting with the patient.
- Support the patient's confidence in his physician, even when they have little personal faith in the particular practitioner.
- Present a positive outlook to the patient concerning his condition and its likely outcome or toward his ability to cope with the resultant state.
- Establish good rapport and positive interpersonal relationships with all patients.
- Encourage the patient to express his feelings.
- Treat the patient as a whole person instead of as just so many body parts, systems, or diseases.

- Tell the patient what they will do before they do it.
- Work within the constraints of asepsis, accurate patient identification, and coverage by physician orders where required.
- Base actions on knowledge of pathology and the human body and its responses to illness and therapy.
- Carefully monitor the patient's condition, reporting critical changes to the physician as well as using them in nursing decisions.
- Provide body hygiene and implement therapies dictated by the physician or by knowledge of the patient's condition.
- Preserve the functional capacities of the patient's body.
- Work toward the patient's return to health with optimal retention of capacities or toward a peaceful and dignified death.

The next set of premises have to do with the nurse's beliefs, values, and expectations. Nurses believe that:

- They should feel empathy, not sympathy, for patients.
- The patient should acquiesce to their care.
- Cleanliness is important.
- They should suspend judgment of the patient, whatever his life-style and background.
- They should support the patient's inherent dignity.
- Illness and accidents, with the exception of some related to life-style, happen to people serendipitously and are not their fault.
- They take ultimate responsibility for their own actions, even for acts done under physician's orders.
- Nursing is an art and a science.
- Nursing is a separate, independent profession.
- They have a moral obligation to their patients above all others.

This is not to say that nurses always act on these premises. But when they break one, they are conscious that they are doing something irregular. They probably pause to reflect and justify the deviance to themselves, if not to others.

ANALYZING THE INHERENT THEORY

If one assumes that these premises represent a theory of nursing, how might one analyze them as a coherent framework? Obviously they represent a helter-skelter set of values, rules for action, and expectations—an ad hoc collection (descriptive theory) at best.

One way to analyze a theory is to explore the separate theory parts. One of the most arresting things about these premises is the mixed values concerning honesty—authenticity, if one prefers the existential term. There are pleas for honesty (the patient should be told his condition and prognosis, allowed to vent his feelings) right along with masking of the nurse's own feelings (denial of the nurse's repulsion for certain sights, smells, tasks; denial of embarrassment on the part of the nurse; inculcation of empathy instead of sympathy). There may be outright dishonesty on the nurse's part in supporting the patient's faith in the physician, pretending confidence whether or not the nurse feels it.

It is inconsistent for a theory to support values of honesty and dishonesty simultaneously. Interestingly, the honesty is required from the patient, the dishonesty from the nurse. The bifurcation of values may be intellectually irresponsible when different values and goals are held for half the population (patients) than for the other half (nurses).

Our normative theory of nursing, incidentally, is not irrevocably open to the criticism that a schism exists between patient and nurse. It *is* possible to envision a single race of persons in which half are honest and half selectively dishonest. Nonetheless, it is a peculiar state of affairs at best.

Perhaps the most gracious thing that can be said about the deceptions advocated on the nurse's part is that they are aimed at making a difficult experience easier for the patient. An existentialist, of course, might find such deception difficult to justify. Some theories of nursing claim to be based on existential principles advocating authenticity and honesty on the part of the nurse as well as the patient. Sometimes existential theories are advocated without considering how they conflict with present nursing practices. Consider the two conversations below, the first from the normative theory of nursing, the second from an existential perspective.

Normative example:

PATIENT: I'm sorry you have to do that, nurse. Irrigating a colostomy is revolting.

NURSE: It doesn't bother me at all, Mr. Smith; it's part of my job. I do this every day. You'll get used to it soon, and it won't seem so bad.

Existential example:

PATIENT: I'm sorry you have to do that, nurse. Irrigating a colostomy is revolting.

NURSE: It's distasteful, but it has to be done. Once you're used to it, it won't be quite as unpleasant.

In most cases, the second example would be more honest, but even the nurse who claims to want authentic, existential relationships with patients, may—because of indoctrination in the norms of nursing—have difficulty in being true to her principles. Yet a consistent existential perspective does not call for authentic behavior only when convenient.

The dictate that approves of empathy but not sympathy is a related aspect of the normative theory. The advice may be symptomatic of other distancing tactics recommended to the nurse (eg, masking disgust or embarrassment). Even the nurse's uniform and professional status may be seen as distancing strategies. There is a tension between creating distance from the patient versus establishing rapport (another dictate of the normative theory). It is unlikely that both can be achieved simultaneously. Which is best? Which is healthy? For whom—the patient or the nurse? In demanding both distance and closeness simultaneously, the normative theory can be accused of holding incompatible elements.

Every theory of nursing must deal with two sorts of people: patients and nurses. The nature of this bifurcation is important in analyzing any theory of nursing. Indeed, some theories are contrived as if the patient and the nurse were creatures from different planets. Take, for example, a theory that explains man (the patient) on a biologic stimulus–response basis, yet describes the nurse as acting out of a psychological, free-will orientation. Such a theory has an unjustified schism. After all, nurses and patients do come from the same root race. If the theory purports that patients operate on the basis of stimulus–response, there is no reason to assume that nurses function on a different principle.

The shift in the nature of the human being between patient and nurse often is more subtle than this illustration. Some theories see the patient in one context, for example, a biologic one, while the nurse is seen in another, the psychological perhaps. Another theory might describe the patient as a person involved in making health care decisions while treating the nurse, simultaneously, as the sole decision maker. Always ask, are the nurse and patient members of the same species, do they function in same world?

Another tension in the normative theory of nursing is that created by the difference between parts and wholes. Much of the education on which nurses base their actions (physiology, pathology, pharmaceutics) is founded on disciplines that compartmentalize the human into parts. Yet nurses are expected to act toward patients in a holistic fashion above and beyond a consideration of parts. Can one learn in one manner, yet act in another?

In the normative theory, there is a clear theme that positive emotions are supportive of health and recuperation (eg, anxiety and pain are bad for the patient; the nurse maintains a positive outlook and offers reassurance, supports the patient's faith in his physician, and suspends judgment of the patient). This endorsement of positive emotions may remind the reader of Norman Cousins's (1979) advocacy of laughter as a cure for disease. To what degree does this aspect of the theory (positive emotions as curative) conflict with the simultaneous reliance on sciences such as pathology and physiology?

Peculiarly, when emotions are examined in nursing curricula (rather than inferred in normative rules), they are seldom explored as healing tools. Emotions are studied as feelings a patient has, not as tools the nurse uses. There is a disjunction between what nurses are instructed to *do* concerning the patient's emotions and what they are taught *about* emotions.

In the normative theory, certain values are accepted with little examination. For example, independence on the part of the patient is always seen as a condition to be promoted. But little research has been done to test for therapeutic effects from periods of dependency.

The aspects of normative theory discussed here are not comprehensive, but they illustrate what happens when we juxtapose various individual components. That's only the beginning of an analysis. Next we'll look at the theory as a whole.

THE THEORY AS A WHOLE

In analyzing any theory, it must be viewed as a conjoined set of elements to be considered in terms of balance and representativeness. One looks for what is missing as well as for what is present. From this perspective, the dictates of the normative theory focus heavily on values and emotive aspects of care.

In contrast, little attention is given to methods. True, one finds obeisance to asepsis and cleanliness, but there is not much that could be termed methodology. For a profession in which much of the practitioner's time is spent in overt, physical action, this is peculiar. The technology of bodily care (or principles directing it) is curiously absent from the list.

Even though most of the values and goals of the theory are emotive, there is little indicating what methods the nurse should use in achieving them. How does one care for a patient *as a whole*? How does one effectively *reassure* a patient? How does one *reduce anxiety*?

Sometimes use of the reflective question (a possible method for achieving patient self-awareness) is included in the premises for the normative theory. In practice, the reflective question often turns out to be a device behind which the nurse hides to avoid answering awkward questions.

The lack of premises concerning methods may not be as surprising as it first appears. More effort has been given to creating taxonomies of nursing diagnoses (intellectual labeling), with less written concerning methods of nursing intervention (practical hands-on care). Taxonomies of nursing interventions have been composed at the University of Iowa and are discussed later in this book.

Of similar interest is the focus on the nurse as monitor. Observing appears to be an important function in the normative theory. But monitoring, like diagnosing, is an intellectual act rather than something *done* to or for the patient. Only one premise in our theory deals with what use the nurse makes of the information gained in monitoring. The linkage between monitoring and action may be an area needing more attention. Indeed, physicians who mentor nurse practitioner students often complain that their actions consist of too many referrals instead of direct action. It may be that this represents an unwanted passivity in the nursing norms.

Another impression of the normative theory comes from the large number of prohibitions it contains. Many dictates concern what nurses should *not* do rather than what they should. Is the focus on the negative disempowering? Several sociologists have commented on this negative aspect in nursing.

Suffice it to say:

1. There is a general consensus concerning what should be done by nurses.
2. The premises can be examined together from a theoretical perspective.
3. They form an inconsistent pattern of ad hoc items, some of which are incompatible with each other.

The list seems to be incomplete in terms of offering guidance regarding *methods* and *hands-on aspects* of nursing care.

Finally, the reader may wish to know that the premises selected for the so-called normative theory were the items most often volunteered by students in numerous graduate education classes. The same exercise with different groups of nurses might have produced different premises. The ones identified here, however, have been consistently identified.

NORMATIVE THEORY UPDATED?

The normative list offered in this chapter accumulated over a decade of asking students to reminisce on their education. Some elements may have fallen by the wayside in the hectic changes of the last few years. For example, cleanliness may no longer be next to godliness. In fact, a patient is lucky to get a bath in many frenzied institutions.

Another change involves blame. In many cases, the patient is made to feel responsible for his disease—more likely, ironically, if it is cancer than if it is alcoholism.

Has the normative theory of nursing changed over the last decade? I propose that nursing can be perceived as taking place through three different modalities of practice, each with its own approach. These modalities most closely relate to the settings in which the care is offered.

Acute Care

In hospitals, nursing has become care of the body. We might think of acute care as the *body shop*. Here, homeokinesthesia is the game. The medical model reigns as nurses and physicians share patients, goals, and ideologies. Despite attempts to substitute nursing theories, on the whole, nurses in hospitals think in the medical model, using differential diagnosis or problematic thought, translating as necessary to chart according to nursing models. (See Chap. 4 for an illustration of this point.)

As patient acuity has intensified in the hospital, the body shop image has prevailed. Intensive monitoring of all body systems is possible and necessary given the heroic therapies used on people. Ongoing adjustments in interactive body systems present a subtle dance of interventions, first with this system, then with that. These body systems are associated with the medical model of man, not with more esoteric nursing theories.

For acutely ill patients, nursing has become medicine, with monitoring/adjusting tasks in which the nurse either makes the adjustments or tells the physician exactly what is required. And the physician, if secure enough, will order what the nurse suggests. In essence, the medical model is alive and well.

With the radical human body insults, the intensive monitoring, and invasive therapy required in the acute care setting, it is not a bad idea for nurses and physicians to be working with the same model. It certainly improves their ability to communicate. Benner, Tanner, and Chesla's (1996) book indicates the interwoven nature of nurse and physician roles. In an emergency situation, having either an expert nurse or an expert physician present may save the day. Differences aside, if no one on the team is at the expert level of practice, the patient may not fare well.

It is most difficult to argue that medicine and nursing are separate and different professions in acute care. Nurse practitioner roles enhance this blurring across the lines. Many nursing schools support the model of nurse as junior physician, whether or not they realize it. In nursing master's level programs, course content is more and more practitioner oriented rather than focused on discrete clinical specialist knowledge.

The truth is that, in this highly technical practice, the caring, interpersonal elements seldom come first in the nurse's mind. Indeed, the old activities associated with aspects of caring (such as bathing and feeding) are often done by bath aides, feeding specialists, and nurses' aides. In acute care today, the registered nurse primarily does advanced procedures, and I suspect that the theory most used is the medical model.

Step-Down Care

The case is different in nursing homes, long-term care facilities, various levels of convalescent care, and home care. The interaction theories, the old public health models, and most extant theories of nursing can still be applied in these settings. Among others, Roy (1989), Orem (1985), problem-solving, man–environment models, and most constellations of the nursing process can be used, and often are, in these settings.

For one thing, the pace is slower—and by that, I do not mean that the case load is lighter. Even when the nurse is swamped, she has time to mull over her care designs. Plus, she has fewer interactions with physicians and other health care workers and more control over her practice world.

The environment for home care and long-term care is similar to what existed in hospitals when most extant nursing theories were being formulated. The care given in homes and extended care facilities today is what used to be offered in hospitals. In these settings, the nurse has the opportunity to think of the whole person; there is the luxury for a more comprehensive view of the patient beyond mere body work.

Whereas the body shop (acute care) was cell/organ/system oriented, step-down level of care is more macroscopic: man in his environment. How does the patient with the recently fractured hip manage at home? Activities of daily living tend to be a major focus; family and community relations get considered. Nurses in step-down environments often use a problem-oriented approach, whether they say so or not. A problematic approach works well in these environments and tends to be compatible with a holistic conceptualization of man. (Both holism and a problem-oriented approach are examined in detail later in this book.)

The step-down care environment is also the home of the middle level nursing theory, partly because these patients tend to be sorted by kind. Geriatric care is a good example. Here reinvolvement theories compete with disengagement theories, and bodily safety takes second place to client peace of mind as quality of life issues modify care practices. The arena of step-down care is exciting because its domains are of more interest to nurses than to physicians—arenas where it is more appropriate to consider the whole person.

Mind–Body Care

The third nursing area deals with what I call mind–body work. Here the nurse works with the well or vulnerable in the community, often in a private practice, in places of employment, or in community settings where groups come to seek enhancement of their health or quality of living. The services offered in mind–body work range from exercise, to smoking cessation, to psychotherapy (often Jungian), to stress reduction. Psychosomatic is definitely not the descriptive word for these services because most of these mind–body ventures focus on wellness.

Nurses in these settings use the expansion, improvement, and development theories, many laying claim to theories of Rogers (1970, 1990, 1994), Newman (1979, 1994), Parse (1981), or Dossey and colleagues (1995). One hears of chakras, energy, therapeutic touch, spirituality, recovery programs, and practices like those of Krieger (1981) and Quinn (1984, 1989, 1992). And—yes—some of the caring theories, such as Watson's (1979, 1988) and Leininger's (1988, 1991), creep in.

In the mind–body work, the theory often is developmental, usually highly personal versus the public health/community orientation of step-down nursing. Psychotherapy, acupuncture, holistic healing, meditation, guided imagery—many newer techniques prevail in this arena. This is where many entrepreneurial nurses cluster, with both clinical nurse specialists and nurse practitioners often in private or collaborative practice.

RELATION OF NORMATIVE THEORY TO NURSING THEORIES

One may speculate concerning how much the normative theory of nursing affects nurses ostensibly using other theories of nursing. We described earlier the difficulties that the normative theory presents for a nurse attempting to act from an existential base. Nor is the existential theory the only one that might clash with the normative theory. Holistic theories often have different notions as well.

The normative theory also conflicts with growing sentiment concerning personal responsibility for disease and illness. Some newer theories claim the individual, on some level, chooses his or her degree of illness or wellness.

Surprisingly, nurses educated using various theories of nursing are still able to work together efficiently and effectively. They are able to evaluate each other's work and generally agree on whose practice is excellent, whose poor. This speaks to some underlying agreement concerning what nursing is all about.

Let us look for a moment at the behavior of two nurses using different theories, those of Orem (1985) and Johnson (1980). Suppose that on sequential days these nurses are assigned to the care of the same patient: a young woman, in deep coma with extensive cranial trauma, on a Stryker frame because of additional spinal cord injuries.

Surprisingly, the two nurses would do just about the same things for the patient, albeit with subtle shadings. Even the shadings, however, might be due to personal style as much as nursing theory. Surely neither would let the patient's eyes remain open without lubrication; neither would neglect skin care; neither would ignore fluid intake and output ratios; neither would allow dependent edema to accumulate in tissues if it could be prevented; and neither would neglect to test for changes in the woman's level of consciousness.

These nurse behaviors are easily explained by Orem's theory of self-care. The nurse using Orem's theory is simply substituting for the self-care the woman would provide for herself if she were able. It is more difficult to justify these actions on the basis of Johnson's theory—a theory in which the nurse intervenes in patient behavioral systems. Indeed, the woman's behavior, so far as we know, is highly limited. This is not to say that Johnson's theory could not be turned and twisted to fit the case; indeed, it could.

The issue is whether the theory is turned and twisted to fit what the nurse perceives needs to be done anyway or whether the theory effectively dictates what she should do. Is the nurse's action dictated by some implicit normative theory? Is the purported theory (Johnson's) simply an overlay?

This is not a criticism of Johnson's theory; in numerous cases Johnson's theory would be an effective basis of care, and Orem's theory would have to be twisted and turned to fit. The issue is whether or not a normative theory of nursing underlies what nurses actually do with patients. If there is such a normative theory, it is time that we define it more adequately. If we could capture the theory of extant practice, we would have an excellent basis for improving it, and it would be a challenge to work with an *is* theory as opposed to an *ought* one.

Another possibility is that, as nursing theories develop, they may become more discrete concerning what nursing acts their followers will perform. Then greater differences in practice may appear than is presently the case. Perhaps, eventually, a customer will select nurses holding one theory over nurses using another the same way he selects today among physician, osteopath, and homeopath.

SUMMARY

Nursing theory should direct a practical set of activities directed toward specific goals. One way to keep our eye on the essential linkage between theory and practice is to periodically examine how nurses practice, asking what tenets, values, and directives undergird what nurses actually do and think. Are these values and directives consistent with those expressed in our formulated nursing theories? If not, either the theories or the practices should be made consonant. Ultimately theory must be reality based if it is to serve us. Looking at the notions that control the practice of any era is a first step in formulating or evaluating theories.

Looking at practice through theory-colored glasses also enables us to see changes from era to era, from one practice setting to another. Behind all examination of extant practice rides the teasing question: Is there an unstated but accepted theory of nursing that is prior to and basic for the theories that are advocated? If so, how can we tease the theory out so that it may be clarified and examined?

PRACTICE EXERCISE

Just as one can derive a nursing theory from familiarity with practice (as was done in this chapter), it is possible to infer a model of nursing from written works that address nursing practice. Select three clinically based articles. (Do not choose articles about nursing theory or sociologic factors of practice.) Read the articles concerning clinical practice through "theory-colored glasses," then describe each writer's theory of nursing. Make a brief list of premises that were stated or could be inferred in each article. Compare and contrast the nursing worlds represented by the papers.

REFERENCES

Benner, P., Tanner, C. A., & Chesla, C. A. (1996). *Expertise in nursing practice: Caring, clinical judgment, and ethics.* New York: Springer.
Cousins, N. (1979). *Anatomy of an illness.* New York: Norton.
Dossey, B. M., Keegan, L., Guzzetta, C. E., & Kolkmeier, L. G. (1995). *Holistic nursing: A handbook for practice* (2nd ed.). Gaithersburg, MD: Aspen.

Johnson, D. E. (1980). Behavioral system model for nursing. In J. P. Riehl & C. Roy (Eds.), *Conceptual models for nursing practice* (2nd ed., pp. 207–216). New York: Appleton-Century-Crofts.

Krieger, D. (1981). *Foundations for holistic health nursing practices: The Renaissance nurse.* Philadelphia: Lippincott.

Leininger, M. M. (1988). *Care: Discovery and uses in clinical and community nursing.* Detroit: Wayne State University Press.

Leininger, M. M. (1991). The theory of culture care diversity and universality. In M. M. Leininger, (Ed.), *Culture care diversity & universality: A theory of nursing* (pp. 5–68). New York: National League for Nursing Press.

Newman, M. A. (1979). *Theory development in nursing.* Philadelphia: Davis.

Newman, M. A. (1994). *Health as expanding consciousness* (2nd ed.). New York: National League for Nursing Press.

Orem, D. E. (1985). *Nursing: Concepts of practice.* New York: McGraw-Hill.

Parse, R. R. (1981). *Man-living-health: A theory of nursing.* New York: Wiley.

Quinn, J. F. (1984, January). Therapeutic touch as energy exchange: Testing the theory. *Advances in Nursing, 6,* 42–49.

Quinn, J. F. (1989, December). On healing, wholeness, and the Haelan effect. *Nursing and Health Care, 10,* 552–556.

Quinn, J. F. (1992, July). Holding sacred space: The nurse as healing environment. *Holistic Nursing Practice, 4,* 26–36.

Rogers, M. E. (1970). *An introduction to the theoretical basis of nursing.* Philadelphia: Davis.

Rogers, M. E. (1990). Nursing: Science of unitary, irreducible, human beings: Update 1990. In E. A. M. Barrett (Ed.), *Visions of Roger's science-based nursing* (pp. 5–11). New York: National League for Nursing Press.

Rogers, M. E. (1994). Nursing science evolves. In M. Mandrid & E. A. M. Barrett (Eds.), Roger's scientific art of nursing practice (pp. 3–9). New York: National League for Nursing Press.

Roy, C. (1989). The Roy adaptation model. In J. Riehl-Sisca, *Conceptual models for nursing practice* (3rd ed., pp. 105–114). Norwalk, CT: Appleton & Lange.

Watson, J. (1979). *Nursing: The philosophy and science of caring.* Boston: Little, Brown.

Watson, J. (1988). *Nursing: Human science and human care: A theory of nursing.* New York: National League for Nursing Press.

4   Basic Assumptions Underlying Current Nursing Practice

IMPLIED THEORY

In the last chapter, we looked at some of the general normative elements of nursing theory. Here we will put this sort of reflection to work in an actual nursing practice situation. Chapter 1 discussed the fact that much nursing theory is based on what ought to be rather than what is. This chapter tries to remedy that.

Extant nursing practice is an interesting place to start because clinical practice is where nursing knowledge is grounded. Nursing knowledge, arising from practice, should shape our theories, and theories, reciprocally, should direct our practice. Theory, knowledge, and practice should fit naturally together, and in most disciplines that happens. If we cannot evolve theories that truly direct practice, then we are wasting time. If a nursing theory is any good, it will be practical.

Not all nurses view nursing theory as a vital component of practice. Perhaps this is because of deficits in our present theories, or it may be an inability on our part to convey the utility of the theories we have formulated. In disciplines that do not admit to having a theory—like medicine—it is interesting to see what occurs when

Much of the material in this chapter was first presented at the Conference on Knowledge Development in Nursing, College of Nursing, Rhode Island University, Kingston, Rhode Island, September 26, 1991.

new ideas conflict with the *implied* theory. American medicine's early resistance to acupuncture is a case in point. Acupuncture meridians ignored known nerve paths, contradicting the cell/organ/system theory that forms the basis of the medical model. No doubt this theoretical incompatibility slowed acceptance of acupuncture despite careful research data showing its effectiveness.

How does nursing theory relate to the actual work that nurses or nursing students do? The last chapter looked at this question from the armchair perspective; the cases illustrated in this chapter arose from my observations and those of my graduate students. I look at extant practice because one must know what is happening *right now*, before saying it needs changing. It is easier to change something one *knows* than to work in a vacuum.

In the last chapter we said no matter what theory a nurse follows, she is likely to do approximately the same things as other nurses when placed in the same situation—and that's truly remarkable. How can so many different nursing theories lead to identical actions? If we were to look at another field—say psychiatry—it does not work that way. A Freudian psychiatrist, a Jungian, and a Skinnerian behaviorist would do very different things with the same client. Their approaches would be unique and their goals distinct.

Yet in nursing, there is much uniformity in the actions of nurses espousing different theories. Do all roads really lead to Rome? Do the different theories and rationales truly result in the same actions? Or with greater development will the various nursing theories prescribe more variation in practice than is the case today? Are our theories rationalizations designed to work backward to a set of acts intuited on a more basic level? Are the nursing theories we have devised actually in service to some overarching but still unrecognized theory of nursing practice?

The descriptive approach, looking at what nurses actually do, has never been popular with nurse theorists. All of our general theories, from Roy (1989) to Orem (1985) to Paterson and Zderad (1988), tell what the good nurse *ought to do*. Despite this strong bias, I assign doctoral students to observe hands-on nursing in various settings—a loose, grounded theory approach. The objective is to have them look at what actually happens and see if they can infer a theory of nursing underlying the practice. Hopefully, they can do this without imposing a ready-made value system on the observations, without being blind to the things one might not *want* to see.

Not every observer approves of what the nurses do, but at least the method offers hope of developing a baseline on nursing practices. In most cases, analysis proves that the nurses were actually working to some end, in some sensible fashion.

STUDENT FINDINGS

I learned a great deal about nursing attitudes in my early work with such observations. I remember, for example, when a class of six doctoral students—each observing independently in diverse settings such as intensive care, nursing clinics, nursing homes, coronary care—all came back with similar findings.

From those observations they wrote a scholarly paper entitled *Avoidance and Distancing: A Descriptive View of Nursing* (Flaskerud, Halloran, Janken, Lund, & Zetterlund, 1979). What impressed this particular group of students was the fact that all the nurses observed used strategies to build space between themselves and their patients. The approach the students took to analyze this behavior was the one we used in class. We asked: If the nurses create space between themselves and their patients, what function does this behavior serve?

So much is written about the necessity for a close nurse–patient relationship, so little about the function that distancing serves, that it is not surprising that the paper received many negative reviews. Indeed, most of the major nursing journals rejected the article, usually with rejoinders that nurses should not be distancing themselves from patients. It was a strong message about nursing theory: Do not tell us *what is* unless it matches our ideal expectations. *Nursing Forum* published the article—the only journal that would take a chance.

Over my years of teaching, I have continued with observation groups of graduate students. The nurses they observed never had trouble identifying the dictates of their nursing practice. Ask the right question at the right time, and nurses can explain why they did X instead of Y or Z. Often these operating dictates had little to do with espoused nursing theory.

PERSONAL OBSERVATIONS

This section describes a time when I personally observed a student nurse at practice. I have no reason to think the day was atypical. My account gives an overview of the relationship of theory and nursing practice as it occurred that day.

The senior student nurse I observed was assigned to a medical unit of a typical acute care hospital. She came on duty at 7:30, heard report from the head nurse, and was assigned to two patients. The first, Mrs. Jones, was a woman of 68 who had suffered a myocardial infarction 5 days earlier. She had been released from the coronary care unit a day ago and was still on cardiac monitoring. In this hospital the monitor could be read from the patient's room or the nurses' station.

The second patient, Willie, had cirrhosis of the liver and had gone into renal failure. He had been on the unit about a week, was on intravenous fluids with more or less normal output, but was still receiving peritoneal dialysis every 6 hours. The problem with Willie, so the head nurse said, was that the doctors wanted to get him off vasopressors, but every time they tried, his blood pressure dropped. At present they were trying again to maintain his blood pressure by an intravenous drip of normal saline, without vasopressors.

I was interested to see that the head nurse called one patient Mrs. Jones and the other Willie. The student nurse adopted those labels, so I will use them here to retain the flavor of the day. While Willie received the lion's share of the nurse's attention, I had no doubt that the name differences reflected an unrecognized social bias.

Both Mrs. Jones and Willie received various medications, by mouth for Mrs. Jones, intravenous for Willie except for a vitamin, which he swallowed. The student checked on Willie first. He seemed to be sleeping but when she talked to him, he opened his eyes and answered coherently. When she quit asking questions, he drifted back into a mild stupor. She took his blood pressure; it was in the low nineties. She immediately went to the head nurse to report it. The head nurse said, yes, it was low, but they were trying to wean him from vasopressors—just watch it and try to stabilize the pressure by regulating the intravenous fluids.

The student went back to the room, speeded up Willie's intravenous drip, then looked at his output bag. Obviously, it occurred to her that if she ran the fluid too fast, Willie would diurese, defeating the purpose of building up blood volume to increase blood pressure. She slowed the drip a little, making it slightly faster than it had been when she first entered the room. While we did not discuss her action, I am certain that her knowledge of the interplay of fluids with the body systems was the source of this correction.

This was the start of the balancing game of the day—to keep Willie from going into shock because of low blood pressure, to keep him from diuresing, yet avoid administering the vasopressors that would lend artificial support to the blood pressure. The student watched Willie like a hawk—his vital signs, his level of consciousness, his blood gases and oxygenation. It was a fine act in achieving equilibrium, and she adjusted the intravenous flow time after time. Several times, she notified the head nurse as the pressure slowly but surely fell. Each time, the head nurse said simply to keep watching it.

The student's attention to Mrs. Jones involved giving her pills.

(Both patients had been bathed by a night bath team.) The student asked Mrs. Jones if she had any pain, and Mrs. Jones said, "Yes, the small of my back is killing me."

The nurse nodded and said, "Let's change the angle of the bed and see if that helps." She cranked the bed up a notch or two. I think it is safe to say this was a token effort more than an expectation that it would bring relief. If the patient had complained of heart pain, I am certain the student's efforts at pain relief would have been more serious. The student did not ask Mrs. Jones any other questions once she knew the patient had no heart-related pain. She reassured Mrs. Jones that she would be available, "if you need anything."

She then checked to make certain the cardiac monitor was attached and working. In truth, the machine monitored Mrs. Jones while the nurse monitored Willie. The student nurse made no attempt to increase her involvement with Mrs. Jones, but then her mind was on the balancing act with Willie. I am certain that the situation would have been different if Mrs. Jones had any symptoms of heart failure.

The student was particularly worried about Willie's status when she let the peritoneal dialysate run into the abdomen. While the fluid was indwelling, she checked his blood pressure every few minutes and again when the fluid was released. Ironically, the only time all day that the nurse relaxed was when the physician finally ordered vasopressors. This did not occur until Willie's blood pressure drifted into the low eighties. Once medication was given, Willie's blood pressure immediately went up to 110, and the nurse breathed a sigh of relief. The only time the student was at ease all day was when the physician admitted failure and resorted to drugs. This served as a humbling reminder that what is best for the patient is not always best for the nurse.

Then what? At the end of the shift, the student—who had been recording medications, treatments, and vital signs all day—went to a well worn, xeroxed copy of nursing diagnoses hanging on a chain in the nursing station. She leafed down until she found a couple of diagnoses that would allow her to say the things she wanted to write. She put the diagnoses into the nurses notes, followed by her comments. She did not go through the rest of the list to see if there were any other diagnoses she should have addressed. Nor had she consulted the list in planning or executing her day's work.

In charting on Mrs. Jones, she did not mention the back pain of which the woman had complained three times during the day. The last two times, the nurse had said, "that happens when you're in bed this many days." The nurse then went off shift to a clinical conference with her instructor. At this conference, they discussed the student's patients based on Watson's carative theory of nursing (1988), the model used by that particular school.

Conclusions

So what is the point? This student ran into two theoretical structures for nursing that day. Let's look at the school's theory of caring. Had the student acted out of that model? Well, she gave care in two senses. First, she was *careful* in monitoring both bodies. True, she relied on the cardiac monitor for Mrs. Jones, but that left her free for the more complex monitoring required by Willie. Yes, she was careful in the sense of cautious or guarding—but that is not exactly Watson's notion of caring. The nurse also expressed care in the sense of *taking care of*, in that she followed medical orders, gave pills, ran dialysate, recorded vital signs. Yet this is not the primary sense of caring in Watson's theory either. One might debate whether she *cared* about either patient in the aspect of care called concern, emotive affect—the notion closest to Watson's theory.

It was clear that the student turned Mrs. Jones aside with platitudes rather than seeking a real relief for her back pain. Yet what would the student have done if Mrs. Jones sensed a willing ear and unloaded her anxiety? The student really was not free to be with Mrs. Jones in that caring sense. (I realize this is casting the student's performance in the best light possible, and she could be faulted for ignoring the patient's back discomfort, let alone discouraging the conversation that might have surfaced with the slightest probing.) But the student's mind was constantly with Willie. It might have been worse if she had offered tidbits of false interest to Mrs. Jones when she was not prepared to follow up on them.

Did she express caring concern for Willie? When she was about to do anything, she always told him clearly, and he looked up from his mild stupor and said, "okay." Beyond this, the student showed no overt signs of emotional attachment—no pat on the arm, no squeeze of the hand. Should she have worked harder at expressing her concern—assuming she had it?

I think the clearest concern shown by the student was her fear that Willie's low blood pressure would bring on a major crisis and endanger his life. Yet I suspect that she was far more interested in removing the possibility of this threatening scenario than she was in weaning Willie from reliance on vasopressors.

I was tempted to go to the clinical conference. If the student did not *care*, affectively, for Willie all day long—I am not saying she did not, I just could not see it—I suspect that she expressed plenty of concern when she gave her report to the instructor. I cannot help but think that the caring theory had almost nothing to do with her actions in the clinical arena.

The second brush with nursing theory occurred when the student had to base her charting notes on the hospital's system of nursing diagnosis. The charting format allowed the nurse to chart only after listing a diagnosis to which her comments related. In this particular use of nursing diagnosis, there was a lengthy, battered list from which she might choose. (It was clear that other nurses thumbed the list daily.)

One might say these nursing diagnoses were important to the student's activities except that she never consulted the list until the end of the day. It was a retroactive effort in which the student hunted until she found a diagnosis that would allow her to say what she wanted to say anyway. The diagnosis was in no way directive of her practice; it was a structure into which she crammed her thoughts after the fact. This nursing theory element had an impact on practice, if not the expected one. It became one more obstacle impeding nursing practice—the student could not talk about Willie until she put her thoughts into one of the dictated categories. This does not mean that I am against the use of nursing diagnosis, but I think a *good* theory should have helped the student during the work of the day. A good theory should be practical; it should direct practice.

Did our student practice all day without any theory? I do not think so. I think she had a theory in mind, and I think it was the medical model of cell/organ/system. I do not think it was a bad model given the two patients in her care. The whole problem with Willie was to maintain a delicate balance among failing systems. The patient had deficits in at least three critical systems—renal, liver, and circulatory—not to mention the resultant deficits in his levels of consciousness and cognition. Frankly, if Willie were part of my family, I would prefer that she worry about his systems rather than focus on affective involvement—*if* she had to choose.

What about the second patient? It may well be that Mrs. Jones was ready—even ripe—for a caring relationship. But this student was not prepared to offer it because of the time and attention demanded by Willie. No doubt the care given to Mrs. Jones was minimal, deficient from any notion of comprehensive care. At least the student made sure the cardiac monitor was attached and working. Are there theories that would have allowed the same focus on vulnerable body systems while adding a more sensitive expression of concern? Why did she seem so little affected by the model promulgated in her school? We may decry the medical model, but I think it was alive and well in this particular student's practice that day. It was the only theory that could account for the student's activities that day.

Let's look for a moment at the nursing process, with its conjoined list of diagnoses supposedly directing practice on the unit. Was it truly directive when the nurse worked backward to it, from a medical model orientation?

If an imposed model is not followed, that is not always bad. Nurses are not stupid; given a chance they seek a directive structure that works efficiently. If I did not have faith in their native intelligence, I would not be interested in inferring theory from observed practice. One may argue that the student ignored the unit's theory of practice because it conflicted with her school's carative model. It is true that students often find themselves in this double bind. In the case of this student, that argument would have been more compelling if she had used the carative model, but she did not.

I think it is safe to say that students are wonderfully creative in subverting all curricular and practice-setting impediments that get in the way of their learning and taking care of patients. The question becomes, what do nurses really learn about giving care, and where and how do they learn it? To what degree, if any, are the theories they learn directing or even modifying that care?

Are the caring theories too global? Do they fail to give the nurse a basis for her actions? Does the nursing process/diagnosis formulation suffer from the opposite fault: presenting an overwhelming number of pieces (process steps and diagnoses)? Can the nurse really consider all the available diagnoses, that is, respond to each one that possibly fits a patient?

The nursing student I observed did not use either of these theoretical models. Instead, she worked on a system of differential diagnosis applied to a cell/organ/system notion of the human—in other words, the medical model.

Some might protest that the nursing process is the same as the medical model, but that is not true. When a nurse assesses her patient using nursing process and nursing diagnosis, she is supposed to identify *all* the applicable nursing diagnoses. In contrast, when a physician assesses a patient, she does not run through the latest classification of accepted medical diagnoses, working her way down the alphabet of diseases. "No, the patient doesn't have Addison's disease; no, he doesn't have a brain tumor; nor Cushing's disease; nor dyspepsia either."

The physician does not consider all the possibilities; instead, she works by the method of differential diagnosis—branching logic instead of checking out a whole world of possibilities. Starting with whatever she recognizes as aberrant (the presenting problem), the physician uses a thought pattern something like this: If it is a tumor, is it cancerous or benign? If cancerous, is it operable or inoperable?

If inoperable, is it amenable to therapy A or therapy B? Instead of tracing out all possible diagnoses, she follows a trail of decision-making through a process of operational thought that makes either/or choices at each step, ignoring and dropping other aspects of the model.

In the nursing process model, this is usually not the suggested format. Most who use the process recommend that a nurse start with *all* the applicable diagnoses, implying that the nurse consider the whole model at one time. In this application nursing is giving support to a system of great complexity. Returning to the case of our student, did we foster nursing theories that were interesting but simply did not work? Was the fault in the systems? In the student? In the conflict between models to which she was exposed?

Nurses fall back on systems that work when it comes to actual patient care. This student nurse, if my perceptions were accurate, used a medical model. I would have difficulty asserting that she was wrong, given her assignment.

In most of our nursing theories, we eschew use of the medical model because nursing is trying to prove its independence from medicine. Should we take a fresh look at the medical model? Is it the best choice in certain situations, with certain patients? Can it be modified or adapted to meet nursing requirements? More importantly, is the medical model the hidden model underneath all our rhetoric? The student I observed had learned it somewhere. I am not advocating that nursing return to a medical model, I am simply saying that, like any other proposition, it should be analyzed for its fit and effectiveness in practice. Any theory, including the medical model, should be treated with similar dispassion.

This student's behavior (failing to use models she *ought* to use) was not unlike the situation in which my other students identified the principles of distancing and avoiding. In both cases, unpopular notions reared their heads in actual practice. As long as we let an ingrained value system keep us from examining unpopular notions—like avoidance, distancing, and the medical model—we have not gained the psychic distance necessary for dispassionate evaluation. Something is lacking in our intellectual honesty when the behaviors demonstrated by nurses at work are judged and found wanting before being given due consideration.

Finally, the reader is advised to peruse the work of Benner (1984) and Benner, Tanner, and Chesla (1996) who have done a masterful job of looking at nurses in practice in relation to how they think on the job. This work examines thought processes as they relate to experience and finds that nurses' ways of thinking change over time. For example, the thought processes behind the nursing process may help the nurse with lower levels of expertise while hamstringing the one with more intuitive and higher level expertise.

Should practice become the basis for all theory generation? Not necessarily. But it should not be overlooked as a testing ground for our notions of theory. Some of our best theorists are those who approach their own practice with a questioning manner and an open eye.

SUMMARY

This chapter has discussed the notion that practice and theory should inform each other, that theory should be practical and directive of actual practice. In a brief day's observation, I saw instances of conflict between practice and theory as well as instances where the nurse probably was not aware of the theoretical basis for many of her actions. Although it is easier to see inconsistencies as a "removed" observer, there is no reason why a practicing nurse cannot think about such issues during her own practice.

One of the obstacles to a nurse's thinking about what she is doing is the set of dictates she brings to her work, the set of values and models popular at any historical moment. Differences between the philosophies of a school and a practice arena may place a special burden on nursing students. This problem deserves serious attention by faculty and practicing nurses in clinical settings where students are expected to perform.

REFERENCES

Benner, P. (1984). *From novice to expert: Excellence and power in clinical nursing practice*. Menlo Park, CA: Addison-Wesley.

Benner, P., Tanner, C. A., & Chesla, C. A. (1996). *Expertise in nursing practice: Caring, clinical judgment, and ethics*. New York: Springer.

Flaskerud, J. H., Halloran, E. J., Janken, J., Lund, M., & Zetterlund, J. (1979). Avoidance and distancing: A descriptive view of nursing. *Nursing Forum, 2*, 158–174.

Orem, D. (1985). *Nursing: Concepts of practice* (3rd ed.). New York: McGraw-Hill.

Paterson, J., & Zderad, L. (1988). *Humanistic nursing*. New York: National League for Nursing Press.

Roy, C. (1989). The Roy adaptation model. In J. Riehl-Sisca, *Conceptual models for nursing practice* (3rd ed., pp. 105–114). Norwalk, CT: Appleton & Lange.

Watson, J. (1988). *Nursing: Human science and human care: A theory of nursing*. New York: National League for Nursing Press.

5 Touch or Technology: A Tension in Today's Nursing Theory

DICHOTOMIES IN NURSING

At present, one of the tensions in nursing theory is a standoff between two highly disparate philosophies. The two camps can be captured in Naisbitt's (1982) coining of the opposing ideologies of high touch and high tech. In the practice environment, be it hospital, home care, or long-term care facility, growth is toward increasingly high-tech practice. In contrast, many entrepreneurial nursing practices and educational programs are dominated by high touch, often with programs centered around one or another theory of caring or a holistic conception of man.

In the complex, highly demanding acute care setting, there are times when practicing nurses may feel too pressured to tend to the patients' needs for human concern (high touch in Naisbitt's terms). The pressures of downsizing of nursing staff add fuel to such feelings by creating role overload and resentments. Some nurses cope by tending the machines rather than the patients.

Given the complexity and high demands of the intricate life-preserving/monitoring machinery in acute care, it is easy to understand this failing. Coping by distancing, we would say, if a patient did it. At its worst then, high tech may be a flight from the emotive demands of an environment in which patients are sicker and sicker, technology ever increasing, at the same time that nursing resources are stretched thinner and thinner. Hospitals and large care organizations try to combat this withdrawal by programs designed to instill a customer orientation.

It is not surprising that some practitioners have taken the flight from this technical complexity. One tactic is a flight *to* something perceived to be better, for example, practice in one of the many newly developed nonacute care settings—ambulatory care, community facilities, long-term care, and other subacute facilities. In schools of nursing, the movement into alternate care settings from the hospital is engendered by two circumstances: a commitment to a distributive pattern of nursing and a failure to find adequate clinical experiences available in the shrinking acute care settings. In other cases, movement to low technology is a flight *from* something regarded as fearsome. Overwhelmed by the machines, by the rapid turnover of procedures and equipment, uncertain of how such complex and changing practices can ever be taught or learned, some nurses have selected to practice through theories that do not address the increasing technology of health care. On the positive side, other nurses have a conviction that nursing is not about the high technology of acute care and that it should be located in a more comprehensive perception of humans.

Such theories may incorporate a spiritual component of man; they may see the human being as an entity that is far more than physiology. In other cases, the theories are located in nursing's caring domain, that is, in affect and emotion rather than technology.

This is not to call holistic or caring theories inadequate. The truth is that the needs for high tech and high touch are both present in many care-giving environments. The philosophic problem is that these two notions seldom rest comfortably within the same theory.

In light of the passage of time, it is interesting to go back to the origin of high tech/high touch as coined by Naisbitt (1982). By now, most people have adopted his terms but forgotten what he said about them. Naisbitt forecast the dichotomy but saw the technology as inevitable, unstoppable. High touch, he said, would develop as a rebellion to it:

> *A poignant example of what I mean by high tech/high touch is the response to the introduction of high technology of life-sustaining equipment in hospitals. We couldn't handle the intrusion of this high technology into such a sensitive area of our lives without creating some human ballast. So we got very interested in the quality of death, which led to the hospice movement, now widespread in this country. (p. 42)*

It is clear that nurses and other health care workers have created backlash movements as Naisbitt predicted. This does not mean that these backlash movements lack inherent value. No one would deny the importance of the hospice movement, for example. But that does not lessen the accuracy of Naisbitt's prediction.

REACHING EQUILIBRIUM

What was Naisbitt's solution to the dichotomy between high touch and high tech? He called for a balance, a notion that needs careful consideration. How does one balance high tech/high touch in the modern acute care health care facility? Not by ignoring the machines and teaching only affect, nor by performing high-tech skills with human needs ignored. Naisbitt's solution was *balance*, not an either/or choice. And the higher the technology, the greater the need for compensating high touch. This problem is not yet solved by most extant nursing theories. A patient wired to three beeping machines in an intensive care unit is more in need of high touch than is the patient receiving less technologically imposing care. Striking the right proportion requires excellence in both domains simultaneously. The caregiver must have the technological skills *and* the human element of caring. Neither alone is adequate. The truth is that increased technology has not only made the techniques of nursing practice more complex, but it has also made the need for high touch more intensive.

NURSING THEORIES: BLENDING HIGH TOUCH, HIGH TECH?

In theoretical terms, a problem arises when trying to serve goals of high touch and high tech simultaneously. The problem is that these two notions typically arise in competing ideologies about the world and the patient (ie, in the context).

The patient for whom high tech is applied is primarily viewed as a physical body, expected to react like most other bodies. The neurologic, chemical, and physical aspect of body are the targets of the high-tech strategies. The therapeutic interventions are designed to bring these elements of being into conformity with desired norms. The nurse practitioners in most of my classes are concerned with these technological elements of care.

In contrast the patient for whom high touch is applied is the individual in his personhood, the human being separate from all other persons. High touch concerns the person as he expresses his unique needs, desires, will, and emotions. These aspects of personhood clearly affect health but cannot be programmed; they are not amenable to high-tech intervention.

Biofeedback might be considered a technique that, to some degree, bridges from person to body, from high touch to high tech, because it uses the mind to influence the body. Similarly, some uses of imagery may cross the line. Consider the case in which a patient with cancer is told to imagine his healthy cells destroying the aberrant ones. The general consensus now is that such imagery is effective.

Often nursing theories attempt to address both person and body, touch and technology. The issue is whether they do it effectively or whether they address two contexts instead of one. Consider Levine's early theory (1971). Conservation of energy and structural integrity dealt with man as biology, whereas conservation of personal and social integrity dealt with man as a person. But the issues are cast on two different playing fields. In her later work, Levine (1973) attempts to bridge this contextual difference by applying homeokinesis to both aspects of man, but the disjuncture is still evident.

The popular nursing process, and its related taxonomy of nursing diagnoses, favors the high-tech side of the equation even though some of the diagnoses are psychological or sociologic in nature. The greatest "selling point" of the process has been that it is so scientific that it is "removed" from the personhood of the nurse. Supposedly, any group of intelligent nurses studying the same patient would come up with the same diagnoses. The system calls for application to all patients of routinized assessment tools (the patient's history, physical examination) to reveal self-evident conditions. The assumption is that the diagnoses are logical conclusions, external to the nurse, conclusions that are *in fact* evident in the patient.

This removed, research-directing theory contrasts with notions of nursing arising from the caring and holistic models. In these models, the personhood of both nurse and patient is involved, making human interactions unique, not replicable. In most of the caring theories, caring is an emotion the nurse brings to the situation by virtue of how she feels, not a tool she carries with her like scissors.

Nursing's move toward caring and holistic theories could be seen as a reactive stroke to the high tech of our provider environments— just as Naisbitt predicted—except for the positive goals of these theories. Nevertheless, successful nursing depends on blending and balancing high touch and high tech in equal measure, and we must find a way to bridge these opposites in our nursing theories. Dossey presents one of the few nursing theories that begins to bridge holistic and physiologic approaches by finding the linkage between mind and body reactions. As Dossey (1995) says:

> . . . *perception (or imagery) elicits mental and emotional responses that generate limbic, hypothalamic, and pituitary biochemical responses; in turn, these biochemical responses bring about physiologic changes that are perceived and responded to, completing a cybernetic feedback loop (p. 95)*

Dossey is one of the first to base an holistic theory of nursing on a physiologic explanation. She recounts mind modulations with the autonomic nervous system, the endocrine system, the immune system, and the neuropeptide system. The implications she draws follow:

> *It is clear that the autonomic, endocrine, immune, and neuropeptide system within our bodies can communicate with each other. This information helps us understand the reasons that holistic nursing interventions such as relaxation, imagery, music therapy, touch, and meditation are so effective. The therapies are grounded in science. Our challenge is to refine the processes and techniques for specific modulation of bodymind symptoms within nursing practice. (p. 107)*

Hence, we find Dossey beginning a theory that can rationally bind high touch and high tech through, what she labels, a "bodymind linkage."

THEORIES OF TOUCH

Touch, itself, has become an important value in nursing and is worth pursuit as the origin of many middle level theories. At first glance, touch would appear to be the same as Naisbitt's high touch, but the situation is not that simple. Naisbitt's concept of high touch concerns caring more than physical contact. Touch, as used in nursing, however, usually involves the physical contact of nurse and patient. Weber (1990) identifies several discrete notions of touch: to be in contact with, to communicate, and to lay hands on.

The first meaning (contact) represents a physical-sensory model, typical of an Anglo-American philosophy, Weber says. The second (to communicate) is associated with European existential and phenomenological models, whereas the last (laying on hands) comes closer to a field model and possibly an Eastern philosophy.

Nursing has done research on touch in all three of these paradigms. Diamond (1990, p. 73) explored the thesis that tactile stimulation improves central nervous system function. Discussing mammalian forebrain responses to varied environmental conditions of touch, the author documents chemical and structural modifications in nerve cells. Diamond's work illustrates Weber's first sort of touch: a physical-sensory model. This meaning of touch crosses the line into the high-tech ideology. Diamond talks about nerve cells, not persons; stimuli and responses, not human values or perceptions.

Weiss's (1991, p. 34) work also focuses on the physical-sensory model (with some crossover to other ideologies), evolving a model interrelating qualitative and quantitative dimensions of touch, including location of touch divided into 19 body areas, actions divided into 28 gestures, duration measured in seconds, intensity measured in four levels, and frequency of contact within specified time frames.

Much of the work on touch in nursing resides in Weber's second ideology, a phenomenological meaning, where touch is seen as human communication. Consider Fanslow's (1990) discussion of the elderly:

> *The human need for touch on all these levels does not lessen as we grow, develop, and age. Rather, the need for touch on all levels increases with age and wisdom. Physical, psychological, and emotional touches are all essential for the proper establishment of internal sources of security, self-image, trust, and interdependence. (pp. 542–543)*

In this view touch is both bodily and mental. Sympathetic communication and meaning pervade Fanslow's notion.

Therapeutic touch is an example of Weber's final category, with Krieger (1981, pp. 146–147) the first name among nurses in this particular ideology. Therapeutic touch is seen as having a direct effect on the human field through the manipulation of energy. Krieger sees therapeutic touch as having the potential for cure as well as for care.

To make the domain of touch even more complicated than the three senses defined by Weber (all of which have been incorporated into nursing), Leininger (1988, p. 18) makes us aware that touch also has a social meaning—one that may vary from culture to culture.

As a theoretical construct, touch has been adapted to both high-tech and high-touch philosophies. Work such as Diamond's serves as a bridge between those two worlds. One can touch emotionally as well as physically in our common language. Diamond's work purports a scientific, physiologic need for touch, a need shared by all persons. Leininger represents the opposite pole, showing that touch means different things in different cultures. Like Naisbitt's theory, the ultimate solution will not be either/or but many perspectives.

LOOKING AHEAD

The need for high touch increases as technology expands. From a theoretical perspective, few of our nursing theories handle the two elements of high touch and high tech with equal competency. Achieving high tech and high touch is a major challenge for our era; the answer will require looking at our educational and service practices anew. It will involve questioning and revising old patterns, letting go of some cherished beliefs and strategies.

What can we do to bring high tech/high touch into proper balance in our professional practice? One approach views high touch as contextual, as a caring concern, an attitude of human warmth and sympathy, and attitudes are caught, not taught. If faculty and nursing managers show caring concern in everything they do, the attitude will be assumed and copied by students and staff. In this pattern—high touch as context—it becomes something to be demonstrated in performance, not a subject matter for a lecture.

In this tactic, high touch is an essential part of the background in which care occurs, whether high- or low-tech care. There is no need to increase course hours or work hours to achieve it. Instead, the image of how one behaves is conveyed by teachers and leaders as they go about the other aspects of nursing. High touch does not always require the nurse to sit down at the patient's bedside and talk. Caring can be expressed while her hands are busy with other things. A nurse cannot justify saying, "I was too busy to be caring." Caring should be evident in every aspect of her work, hands-on tasks included. In this interpretation, staff learn that the attitude of caring is an expectation, not something the lack of which may be excused by a harried environment. It occurs simultaneously along with task completion.

Because attitudes are caught, leaders must be careful not to damage the positive attitudes that students bring to the profession. Most students enter nursing to "do good" for people. But many soon learn that affect is less significant than scientific dispassion. Students are covertly discouraged from being warm caregivers when praised only for their scientific rigor—for their success in adopting a scientific, removed, disinterested attitude. This is not to say that the science of our craft should be neglected, but the caring element cannot be discouraged either.

ANOTHER OPTION

If, on the other hand, the caring aspect develops its own "technology," it may be necessary to divide nursing into component specialties rather than preparing a person for all sorts of nursing practice in a single program. If techniques like therapeutic touch require their own schooling, it may be that one profession cannot encompass all that is required. Chapter 3 looked at the differences in care ideologies between acute care, step-down care, and mind–body care. It may be that different sorts of nursing will develop, each specializing in its own techniques. As we move into a distributed health care system, instead of a system designed around acute care, this may be the path of the future.

Some aspects of caring technology are breaking off already in the formation of curricula for healers. Many of the students in these schools and classes are nurses, but this "profession in its infancy" is not developing as a subset of nursing.

SUMMARY

High touch/high tech is one of the dichotomies that has marked the history of nursing. Other dichotomies have included science versus art, technical versus professional, care versus cure, clinical specialist versus nurse practitioner. Sometimes the profession handles a dichotomy by picking one side over the other. The early selling of care over cure was one such historical example. The solution was two edged in that it enabled us to set a clear and precise boundary around the profession, but it limited growth as well.

Sometimes the profession solves a dichotomy by trying to have it all. Where theorists assert that nursing is a science *and* an art, we see this solution in effect. Unfortunately, this solution may become a slogan rather than a carefully determined strategy and rationale. Few nursing theories have successfully explained just how this particular opposite pair (art and science) can be combined. It remains to be seen whether the dichotomy between the nurse practitioner role and the clinical specialist role will be solved by an either/or choice, by both existing simultaneously, or, more likely, by some synthesis of the roles.

We have not always picked the best solution in handling our dichotomies. Sometimes the choice has been narrow or self-serving, but seldom should we throw out one element without carefully considering the consequences. The high-touch/high-tech dichotomy demands a successful resolution. The choice of one side to the exclusion of the other has potential negative consequences for the profession.

REFERENCES

Diamond, M. C. (1990). Evidence for tactile stimulation improving CNS function. In K. E. Barnard & T. B. Brazelton (Eds.), *Touch: The foundation of experience* (pp. 73–96). Madison, CT: International Universities Press.

Dossey, B. M. (1995). The psychophysiology of bodymind healing. In B. M. Dossey, L. Keegan, C. E. Guzzetta, & L. G. Kolkmeier (Eds.), *Holistic nursing: A handbook for practice* (2nd ed., pp. 87–111). Gaithersburg, MD: Aspen.

Fanslow, C. A. (1990). Touch and the elderly. In K. E. Barnard & T. B. Brazelton (Eds.), *Touch: The foundation of experience* (pp. 541–557). Madison, CT: International Universities Press.

Krieger, D. (1981). *Foundations for holistic health nursing practices: The Renaissance nurse.* Philadelphia: Lippincott.

Leininger, M. M. (1988). *Care: Discovery and uses in clinical and community nursing.* Detroit: Wayne State University Press.

Levine, M. E. (1971, June). Holistic nursing. *Nursing Clinics of North America, 2,* 253–264.

Levine, M. E. (1973). *Introduction to clinical nursing* (2nd ed.). Philadelphia: Davis.

Naisbitt, J. (1982). *Megatrends: Ten new directions transforming our lives.* New York: Warner Books.

Weber, R. (1990). A philosophical perspective on touch. In K. E. Barnard & T. B. Brazelton (Eds.), *Touch: The foundation of experience* (pp. 11–43). Madison, CT: International Universities Press.

Weiss, S. (1992, Spring). The tactile environment of caregiving. In *The Science of Caring, 2,* (pp. 32–40). San Francisco: School of Nursing, University of California (school magazine).

6 Nursing: The Care Ideologies

TRADITIONS OF CARING: ONE OF MANY PROPOSED BASES FOR NURSING

Many nurse theorists say that caring is at the heart of the profession. This chapter examines that long tradition. What do our theorists mean by caring when it is used as a hallmark for nursing? How does that stance differ from other theories of nursing? More importantly, how do theories of caring differ from each other?

There is general agreement that nurses are caring people; most are drawn to the profession for that reason. That most act in a caring way is different from asserting that the *act of caring* is at the heart of professional nursing practice. In the last chapter we mentioned two models, the nursing process and the medical model, that would place the locus of nursing in a science of diagnosis based on examination and assessment of the patient's physiologic status rather than in caring.

We also have theories that find the nexus of nursing in other places: Levine in conservation, King in transactional agreement on goals, Roy in manipulating stimuli toward desired responses, and Johnson in the realm of behavior. All of these theorists would wish their nurses to be kind, but that is not the point. All find the moving principles of nursing to be located elsewhere. Caring happens in context, they propose; it is on the side—like french fries. The theories discussed in this chapter support caring as the crux of nursing. Many of the "caring" theorists hold that their theories are more in keeping with the new paradigm, the one that challenges the older scientific model.

DEFINITIONS OF CARING

Nurses disagree concerning just what *caring* means. The ambiguous term, caring (sometimes shortened to care), has at least three discrete meanings. The first has to do with *taking care of* in the sense of tending to another, doing for someone else. Taking care of tends to be expressed in physical acts meeting patient needs. The nurse takes care of the patient in tending to his bodily needs, just as the mother takes care of her infant. Care (or caring) in this sense of the word will be labeled *taking care of.*

Orem's (1985) self-care has this sense to it. In her usage, care is a shorthand word for the doing of requisite tasks. This sort of care is an *activity*. In high tech, the first requirement for a nurse is that she be at ease with the equipment and procedures. Taking care of, in this sense, may be closer to high tech than to high touch; at least it has to do with effectiveness in doing for another.

The second notion of *caring* refers to a concomitant emotion or attitude that occurs in the nurse in relation to the patient. The nurse who *cares* is one who has an emotional investment in the patient's welfare; that is, she cares about him. Caring, instead of taking care of, will be used to indicate the case in which the nurse has a positive, concerned feeling for the patient. This definition of caring is *attitudinal* or *emotive* in contrast to the first meaning that we labeled as an *activity*.

Because it is possible for a nurse to *take care of* a patient with a *caring* attitude, the difference between these two meanings is sometimes lost. Yet the notions are separable intellectually and in practice. It is possible that a nurse might *care* yet fail to *take care of,* as in the concerned nurse who sympathizes with an anxious patient but fails to pick up the clues to his internal hemorrhage. In the opposite case, a nurse might *take care of* a patient's needs, using exacting nursing techniques, while still feeling no real concern for him.

A third sense of care involves *caution*, of *being careful* to do something correctly. This meaning carries a sense of guarding against injury or accident. Here care has to do with caution or precision in one's acts. The word, *careful* seems most appropriate with this notion. Like the last meaning, this one is attitudinal, but it concerns a *mind set* rather than an emotion. All three senses of caring may occur simultaneously. A nurse may take care of a patient, with a caring attitude, while being careful to ensure that she does things in a safeguarding manner.

CONFUSING MEANINGS OF CARE

Confusion among the three meanings of caring was evident from early on in the nursing literature. In a classic theory piece, Kreuter (1957) begins with *caring* but encompasses the notions of *taking care of* and *careful* as well:

> The word "care" has precise meaning. It belongs to the intellect and its root is in "sorrow." Care is not akin to cure. It is more related to "pathos" in that the feelings are touched. When one gives care, the feeling is experienced and responded to by extending oneself toward another. Care is expressed in tending to another, being with him, assisting or protecting him, giving heed to his responses, guarding him from danger that might befall him, providing for his needs and wants with compassion as opposed to sufferance or tolerance; with tenderness and consideration as opposed to a sense of duty; with respect and concern as opposed to indifference. (p. 302)

Kreuter's slippage is a mistake than many others have made. One reason is that all three principles of caring have importance in nursing; hopefully, all three are evinced simultaneously in a nurse's practice.

In a modern discussion, Styles (1982) purposely combines two senses of caring:

> Despite our periodic raillery about the word "nursing" and the perceived stigma attached to this designation, our occupation is well named. Nursing is nurturing, nourishing, fostering, caring. Nursing is caring: both the attitude and the activity. Nursing is caring by promoting health and self-reliance for all. Nursing is caring for those who need to be nurtured in relation to their health status, whenever, as long, as frequently as they need it, until that need is removed or revised by recovery, independence, or death. This caring responds to needs ranging broadly between the extremes of information and incentive for maintaining wellness to emotional support and technical assistance for sustaining life and providing comfort. As nurses, our MOTIVATION is caring; our SERVICES are caring and managing; our fundamental TOOL is knowledge, both tacit and explicit; the PRODUCT of the services is health—its maintenance and restoration to the highest possible level of attainment—and physical and psychological comfort. (p. 231)

Some modern theorists, concerned about cloudy meanings, attempt to operationalize their definitions of caring. Gaut (1986) gives this definition:

> To state these requirements in another way, any action may be described as caring if, and only if, the carer (S) has identified a need for care and knows what to do for X (the one cared for); S chooses and implements

*an action intended to serve as a means for positive change in X; and
the welfare of X or what is generally considered as good for X is used
to justify the choice and implementation of the activities identified as
caring. (p. 78)*

Although Gaut's definition might still give us pause concerning
the exact meaning of caring, her decision to relate caring to competency reveals that she is using the action-oriented, *taking care of*
form. Indeed, this form is easier to capture in an operational definition
because it ends in an overt action.

The emotional/concerned meaning of care is harder to pin down.
Authors seldom analyze the nurse's caring in this emotive form. Nor
is it usually interpreted as an act of will; instead caring is seen as a
predisposition. Gaut, in contrast, calls caring an intentional human
enterprise—in other words, taking care of.

Usually one can rely on an author to mean care as *taking care of*
when speaking about nursing behaviors; after all, it is action oriented.
Even here, we find an exception. Wolf, like Gaut, talks about care as
nurse behavior. When we look at the content of the behaviors, however, it is clear that she is actually identifying representative behaviors that give clues to caring (concern). Wolf (1986) calls this form
of caring attachment:

*When attachment behavior is aroused in stressful circumstances, the
attachment figure, the caregiver, terminates the behavior by touching,
clinging to, or reassuring the person experiencing the threat of loss.
(p. 85)*

These are not behaviors in the usual *taking care of* sense because
they reveal the nurse's concern, her emotional involvement. Wolf
(1986, p. 91) developed a Caring Behavior Inventory, arriving at the
following caring behaviors (the 10 highest ranked): attentive listening, comforting, honesty, patience, responsibility, providing information so that the patient or client can make informed decisions,
touch, sensitivity, respect, and calling the patient or client by name.
Like Gaut, Wolf attempts to operationalize a discrete meaning of
caring, but her job is trickier because she is identifying observable
phenomena that stand as evidence of an affective feeling.

EXTENDED MEANINGS FOR CARING

The meaning of caring is not exhausted in the three prior illustrations.
Morse, Bottorff, Neander, and Solberg (1991, pp. 120–121) identify
five conceptualizations of caring as: a human trait, a moral imperative, an affect, an interpersonal interaction, and a therapeutic intervention. They analyze common care theories on these dimensions.

Swanson (1991, p. 163), working on a middle range theory of caring, identifies these caring concepts (paraphrased here):

1. *Knowing—centering on the one cared for*
2. *Being with—sharing feelings, not burdening*
3. *Doing for—comforting, anticipating, performing competently*
4. *Enabling—informing, generating alternatives*
5. *Maintaining belief—believing in, offering realistic optimism*

One of the challenges in defining care has been to capture the affective responses that reflect caring. This is what both Swanson and Wolf are trying to do. A major bias in caring has always been the promulgation of empathy as opposed to sympathy as a desired nurse behavior. Of course, the meaning of these terms has been manipulated from author to author to enable each to take a preferred position without changing terms.

A study by Boyd and Munhall (1989, p. 65), involving the concepts of reassurance and sympathy, identified the following mechanisms of reassurance (paraphrased here):

1. *Giving factual information*
2. *Providing physical comfort such as holding one's hand, touching, covering with a blanket*
3. *Giving theoretical information (eg, explaining what is "normal")*
4. *Supporting the client's power*
5. *Being present, staying and listening*
6. *Projecting a confident, calm manner*
7. *Crying with the client*

This theory building captures the concept in factual behavior, and makes one wonder how the variable of reassurance relates to affective caring. Boyd and Munhall (1989, p. 64) discovered nurses projecting their own feeling into clients erroneously, seeing the client as a victim of unfortunate circumstances when the client had a different perception entirely.

PERSONAL PERSPECTIVES

I would like to reflect on caring I have observed in the three basic meanings of the term from my personal experiences as a patient and as a family member of a patient. Let me begin with my experiences as a family member. Three private duty nurses stand out in my mind, each coincidentally, exemplifying one meaning of caring.

Nurse A was the *careful* nurse. She did the "orders," no more, no less. She was *careful* not to put herself in legal jeopardy. Everything was done on time, using correct methods (technologically advanced care was required). She made no attempt, however, to relate to the conscious patient although she did identify herself and say what she was about to do before doing it. She saw no patient problems; yet as a family member, I could identify many. She made no adjustments in the care plan, established no rapport. In my judgment, *careful* alone simply was not satisfactory.

Nurse B was oriented toward *taking care of*, yet her motivations seemed to be intellectual, not affective. She was fussy about the professional markers; she liked to be called, Miss B, protested when the patient used her first name (visible on her name tag). This nurse did everything that was ordered with great proficiency. In addition, she searched for and remedied patient problems, seeming to enjoy the problem-solving activity for its own sake. Her taking care of included the aspect of being careful without focusing on it. She did all the right things.

She was particularly good at negotiating working arrangements with an obstreperous patient. Her professional judgments were the best of the group discussed here. What she lacked was any sense of caring. I sensed this and so did my sick family member.

Nurse C, in contrast, focused on *caring* in the affective sense. She really cared about the patient. She was not nearly as professional as Nurse B: she used her first name, wore a red sweater and moccasins, and was overweight. When she was not busy, she read *Cosmopolitan* or *Redbook*, but she saw and solved many patient problems because she was sensitive to the patient's reactions.

Some might dispute her professional judgments. She let an exhausted patient sleep, putting off blood pressure checks despite known erratic fluctuations. If she had asked me, I would have made the same decision, and it would have been motivated by the same thing: an emotional response to the patient in addition to an assessment that he needed sleep.

My conclusions about caring based on these observations were simple: the effectiveness of the nursing act was greatly enhanced in Nurse C, who really cared about the patient. From a patient and family perspective, it mattered more than any other factor.

My own experience as a patient was more complex. The nurse who was most supportive, most caring in getting me through a serious life-threatening episode—and I truly felt her support as invaluable—was also the nurse who made serious errors, considerably increasing the pain I would subsequently experience. The caring? It mattered a lot. The errors in therapeutics? That mattered a lot too.

Can caring be the basis of care? In my own mind, I return to the dilemma faced in the last chapter. Care or technology? Can one have dominance? Perhaps the question is which matters most if both are given in competent measure.

THEORISTS ON CARE

Wiedenbach (1970) was one of the early theorists to appreciate the place of caring in nursing. She believed that the intention of the nurse was an important part of her effectiveness, that the same act done with caring and without caring could have a different outcome:

It is the nurse's way of giving a treatment, for example, that enables a patient to benefit from it, not just the fact that a treatment is given him; and it is her way of expressing her concern—not just the fact that she is present or speaks—that enables him to reveal his fears. The nurse's way of using the means available to her to achieve the results she desires in her practice is an individual matter, determined to a large degree, by her central purpose in nursing and the prescription she regards as appropriate to its fulfillment. (p. 1062)

Thoughts and feelings, including reactions, are integral parts not only of what we do or say but also of how we do it. . . The thoughts and feelings that precede and accompany each act are the less apparent parts of nursing; yet, because they set direction for each act, they are the real determiners of the results the nurse achieves. (Wiedenbach, 1963, p. 54)

Wiedenbach (1963) analyzed the "invisible" act of caring, and found it to be a tool that ensures the nurse's successful practice.

The secret of the helping art of nursing lies in the importance the nurse attaches to her thoughts and feelings and the deliberate use she makes of them as she observes her patient, identifies his need for help, ministers to his need, and validates that the help she gave was helpful. If she recognizes her thoughts and feelings, respects their importance, and disciplines herself to harness them to her purpose and her philosophy, not only will she enrich her nursing practice, but she will in all probability experience enduring satisfaction from the helping service she has rendered. (p. 57)

What Wiedenbach calls *concern* is what we label caring. Although she explores these feelings methodically—scientifically, if you will—this is not the way we usually think about the caring part of nursing. Rawnsley (1980) makes a more modern plea in terms not unlike those of Wiedenbach:

If the nurse is to focus on the person rather than the syndrome, however, she must develop a healthy symbiosis of the art and science of nursing within herself. This calls for her to integrate cognitive, psychomotor, and affective skills in such a way that each contributes to and acts in the service of the others, while maintaining its own distinct properties. Identifying, learning, and eventually synthesizing the continually expanding base of knowledge and skills specific to each dimension constitute the science of nursing. The art of nursing consists of successfully

incorporating all three dimensions in practice, as demonstrated in help-
ing behaviors on behalf of patients. (p. 244)

Like Wiedenbach, Rawnsley uses the term *concern* in discussing
caring. For Rawnsley, this concern is nursing's primary business.
Adopting Wiedenbach's notion that the affective component can become a tool, she asserts that there is a science of affect. As she says,
"Yet we must comprehend the affective dimension in order to use
it deliberately" (Rawnsley, 1980, p. 245). Although some might consider these affective aspects instinctive (and unlearnable), Rawnsley
envisions their use in a disciplined fashion, that is, as the science
of the art of nursing:

To relate to the emotional life of others, one must grasp the variety, the
mystery, and even the contradictions intrinsic to the human condition.
Perhaps awareness of this complexity is intuitive; and perhaps apprecia-
tion of it can be cultivated under certain prescribed learning conditions.
(p. 245)

In her attempt to make a science of the emotional side of nursing,
Rawnsley identifies two affective concepts: promotive tension
arousal and empathy. The first is tension coordinated to another's
goal attainment. Helping, according to Rawnsley, is a function of
the level of discomfort or tension a potential helper experiences
witnessing the plight of another. Empathy, she sees as a vicarious
emotional response to the perceived emotional tone of another, a
transient internalization of what it is like to be the other without
being overwhelmed by the identification—in her words, metafeeling
(Rawnsley, 1980, p. 245).

Rawnsley's strategy, to some degree, is to intellectualize feelings,
and this may be a tricky endeavor. Can the emotional response survive under the microscope? Although Rawnsley strives to make a
science of the emotions, Ellis (1969) points out the dangers of losing it:

There is some danger of neglecting, or even rejecting, some of the tradi-
tional, familiar components in nursing as we grow in our emphasis on
science and research. One such component might be what is termed
TLC—"tender loving care." This something or this concept, which some-
one (it would be fascinating to know who) has tried to capture by a
phrase, is nonscientific. We are not likely to do research on it. We do
not have tools to measure it. Yet many nurses, as well as nonnurses,
recognize it as an essential component in nursing for many patients.
(p. 1438)

A New Paradigm Orientation

Watson's (1988) theory is closely associated with the notion of caring.
She holds that, "Caring is the essence of nursing and the most central

and unifying focus for nursing practice" (p. 33). She also says that, "Care and love are the most universal, the most tremendous, and the most mysterious of cosmic forces; they comprise the primal and universal psychic energy" (p. 32). Yet she admits that some persons are caring, others uncaring, defining an uncaring person as:

> . . . *insensitive to another person as a unique individual, nonperceptive of the other's feelings and does not necessarily distinguish one person from another in any significant way. (p. 34)*

Stressing nursing's tradition of caring, Watson (1988) defines caring as a transpersonal value. She gives us a sense of how it feels when caring is present and a taste of its absence as well:

> *It is not so much the what of the nursing acts, or even the caring transaction per se, it is the how (the relation between the what and the how), the transpersonal nature and presence of the union of two persons' soul(s), that allow for some unknowns to emerge from the caring itself. (p. 71)*
> *. . . the degree of transpersonal caring (in this sense of unity of feeling) is increased by the degree of genuineness and sincerity of the nurse. If the recipient feels that the nurse is contriving the feelings and is "going through the process," trying to act upon the other's feelings, and does not feel within his or her self what longs to be expressed, resistance immediately springs up. (p. 69)*

Watson appears to assume the nurse will be a caring person. Perhaps it is a matter of degree, for other parts of her books stress ways to teach better caring through helping the nurse to develop as a person. A good question for Watson would be whether or not applicants to her program are assessed for caring potential before being admitted. One might think this criterion more important than the grade point average if her theory is to be applied consistently.

With her commitment to caring, Watson (1979) calls her theory content/process items, (nurse behaviors) *carative* factors:

1. The formation of a humanistic-altruistic system of values
2. The instillation of faith-hope
3. The cultivation of sensitivity to one's self and to others
4. The development of a helping-trusting relationship
5. The promotion and acceptance of the expression of positive and negative feelings
6. The systematic use of the scientific problem-solving method for decision making
7. The promotion of interpersonal teaching-learning
8. The provision for a supportive, protective, and (or) corrective mental, physical, sociocultural, and spiritual environment

9. The assistance with the gratification of human needs
10. The allowance for existential-phenomenological forces
    (pp. 9–10)

Watson's list of carative factors escapes the three senses of caring previously described in this chapter because it includes aspects that can best be considered as character forming for the nurse. Indeed, it would fit better into the categories of caring identified by Hutchinson and Bahr (1991, pp. 85–88) in relation to the elderly: protecting (safety and surveillance), supporting (facilitating copying and normality), confirming (recognizing personhood), and transcending (prayer and spiritual focus). Hutchinson and Bahr were describing caring behaviors of residents, not nurses, when they arrived at these categories.

Watson (1988) focuses heavily on the spiritual, subjective aspects of both nurse and patient:

> *In transpersonal human caring, the nurse can enter into the experience of another person, and another can enter into the nurse's experience. The ideal of transpersonal caring is an ideal of intersubjectivity in which both persons are involved. This means that the value and views of the nurse, though not decisive, are potentially as relevant of those of the patient. A refusal to allow the nurse's subjectivity to be engaged by a patient is, in effect, a refusal to recognize the validity of the patient's subjectivity. The alternative to caring as intersubjectivity is not simply the reduction of the patient to an object, but the reduction of the nurse to that level as well. (p. 60)*

Watson's theory of caring would be classified as interactional (located, not in the nursing act or the patient, but in the nurse–patient interaction).

In King's (1981) interactional theory, the nurse and patient act, react, interact, and finally transact, that is, agree on a goal or goals. The nature of Watson's interaction is different from King's. Watson's intersubjectivity is transpersonal, occurring in a larger context, beyond both patient and nurse. In this sense we are reminded again of the principle of synergy. The reader interested in a fuller understanding of transpersonal psychology may wish to read Wilber (1979, 1980).

Watson's (1988) focus on the nature of the nurse is intimately tied to her conceptualization of disease as disharmony:

> *Where there is disharmony among the mind, body, and soul or between a person and the world, there is a disjunctive between the self as perceived and one's actual experience, and there is also a felt incongruence with the person, between the I and me and between the person and the world. . . . This incongruence leads to threat, anxiety, inner turmoil,*

*and can lead to a sense of existential despair, dread, and illness. If
prolonged, it can contribute to disease. (p. 56)*

In a theory such as this, treatment of illness takes on a metaphysical, transpersonal character. Caring cannot arise except as an event
between two people:

> *The context for viewing the person and the nurse in the theory of trans-
> personal caring is in the moment-to-moment human encounters between
> the two people. The coming together of the two—one the care-giver and
> the other the recipient—comprise an event. An event connotes an actual
> caring occasion in which intersubjective caring transactions occur. (Wat-
> son, 1988, p. 71)*

Watson is not the only theorist to describe nursing in a new
paradigm, but she is the chief one who focuses on caring as central
to her theory. Watson's later work shifts somewhat, and one could
argue that spirituality replaces caring as the central phenomenon.

A Cultural Orientation

Leininger (1991), another care theorist, at first glance may seem to
be doing the same thing as Watson, but that is not the case. She
considers the patient's world in the sense of the culture in which he
resides. Unlike Watson, her perception of culture is more traditional.
Leininger's patient is affected by whatever world view is held in his
society. If and when a new paradigm is established as mainstream
thought, then she would take that into account.

For now, it serves to call her perspective anthropologic, looking
at the individual as he is influenced by his culture. Her main objective
is to care for the patient, not to reinterpret his world or his meaning
in it. Leininger takes the patient's world as a given and asks how his
perception of it affects on his health and how care should be offered
in light of his perceptions.

What she shares with Watson is that she has fused caring with
another element: in Watson's case, a new paradigm of man and his
existence, in Leininger's case, the patient's culture. As Leininger
(1991) says, "All human cultures had some forms, patterns, expres-
sions, and structures of care to know, explain, and predict well
being, health, or illness status. I held that care was not an isolated
activity . . ." (pp. 23–24). She tightens this notion, making care and
culture indivisible:

> *Culture and care were synthesized as a construct entity that are tightly
> embedded into each other in order to explain, interpret, and predict
> phenomena relevant to nursing. This culture care was conceptualized*

*and transformed into a nursing perspective to develop a body of new
or distinct knowledge in nursing. (p. 24)*

Leininger (1991, p. 37) differentiates folk care systems and professional health care systems, noting that their differences cause problems. The two systems must be linked to avoid culture conflicts,
noncompliant behaviors, and cultural stresses. Nursing, she says,
must consider people's emic knowledge, that is, the meaning their
experiences hold for them. Etic care imposition—based on the caregiver's constructed representation of the empirical world—simply
is not adequate. Leininger (1991) identifies three modes of culturally
congruent care:

1. *Cultural care preservation and/or maintenance*
2. *Cultural care accommodation and/or negotiation*
3. *Cultural care repatterning or restructuring (pp. 41–43)*

These modalities of nursing care incorporate the patient's world
view, including aspects such as: technological factors, religious and
philosophical factors, kinship and social factors, cultural values and
lifeways, political and legal factors, economic factors, and educational factors (1991, p. 43). Leininger's model is complex, but she
makes us sensitive to aspects of parochialism that creep into our
usual theory derivations.

*All too often, some health practitioners do interfere with cultural life-
ways and beliefs of culture by their so-called interventions and lack of
culture knowledge. Hence, the caring nurse generally wants to work with
and be congruent with the norms and values of the culture. (p. 55)*

The vulnerability of Leininger's model is that it requires extensive knowledge of a secondary discipline, anthropology. As Leininger
indicates, the utility of the model depends on the skill of the practitioner in applying it (1991, p. 56). One can argue that merely developing sensitivity to cultural factors—even unknown cultural factors—is an important beginning.

In light of a transcultural perspective, Geissler (1991) takes an
interesting look at the nursing diagnosis work of the North American
Nursing Diagnosis Association (NANDA). She finds the diagnostic
set culture bound.

ANALYSIS OF CARE THEORIES

I find the chief issues, and the chief problems, in care theories arise
when caring (affective) is shifted from context to content or process.
In this fashion, caring becomes, not the *attitude* with which the nurse
delivers her taking care of, but *the* care itself. In essence, the objective

becomes to deliver an affective message of caring. If caring is the basis of nursing, we may have difficulty justifying the fact that nurses also need to learn other things—like regulating body fluids, skin care, and yes, highly technical procedures. When caring becomes the content or the process of a theory, it is difficult to justify the tasks commonly seen as comprising nursing.

The shift of caring into content and process also brings with it a teaching problem. When caring is seen as context, it can be role modeled, caught rather than taught. When it moves front and center as content, then it becomes a subject for study and analysis. Hence affect itself is presented as content to be learned. Will affective caring survive in the nurses's breast if it is held too long under the microscope?

The problems raised above are not meant to negate these interesting theories of caring because it is clear that caring is an important concept in nursing. It is also true that when caring is merely context, it is vulnerable to getting lost. Roberts (1990, p. 69) examines caring in midwifery in an attempt to prove the profession has not been co-opted by the medical model. She finds caring characteristics such as presencing, being with, and virtue alive and well (p. 69). Such important characteristics, she claims, are seldom recognized, rewarded, or taught. It would be difficult to say she is wrong. Clearly, part of the reason these elements get overlooked is that they are less visible as context. Yet many birthing women have shown themselves sensitive to context. Why else select midwives over obstetricians?

Another problem with making caring the central meaning of nursing is that caring is a variable located in the nurse. This is Morse's (1992) criticism, when she suggests that patient-centered variables, such as comfort, are more appropriate. As she says, "This theoretical shift from nurse caring to patient comfort is important, as it changes the focus of nursing research from the nurse to the patient or client" (p. 92). She also finds patient variables easier to measure:

> . . . *patient comfort is both physiologically and psychologically operationizable and measurable. The change in focus permits comfort states to be quantified using indices of individual measures, such as relaxation, recovery, adaptation, coping, or mastery, and incorporates population indices such as morbidity, mortality, and health care costs. (p. 92)*

In an era focused on outcomes, it makes sense to put the most important variables in the patient. Of course, a focus on patient comfort inevitably led to an investigation of, as Morse (1996) calls it, the science of comforting—the comparable nursing principle or act. We might say that comforting brings us back to a notion of caring.

Because they cover such a wide gamut of beliefs and designs, caring theories will probably force nurses to confront and evaluate their own images of the world. Perhaps that is their greatest value. They differ as to: (1) what is meant by caring; (2) whether caring is pure affect or a learned tool; (3) whether caring is an art, a science, or both; and (4) whether caring is tightly bound to another concept (like culture or a new world paradigm).

SUMMARY

Caring is a general term that means many things to many people. At the very least, caring has three discrete meanings: (1) physical acts involved in taking care of; (2) cautionary, protective nurse behaviors; and (3) affective, emotion-laden concern for the patient. Often nurse theorists use the term, caring, without being precise as to which meaning is intended.

Whatever the sense of caring, it is important to know whether it is seen as the *content* of nursing, a *context* in which nursing acts are performed, or a *process* by which nursing is delivered. Even where it is seen "only" as context, caring may have a radical affect on the achievement of nursing goals, as illustrated in Wiedenbach's observations.

In addition to these differentiations, the notion of caring may undergo subtle changes in meaning based on the other concepts in a given nursing theory. For example, where care is linked to culture, the notion is different than where it is linked to a new paradigm view of the world. Because caring is still a popular and value-laden concept, it is important to recognize when it is a mere slogan superimposed on a theory.

Whether the popularity of caring as the dominant principle of a nursing theory will last remains to be seen. Already some authors are recommending its replacement by one or more concepts embedded in the patient, not the nurse. Alternatives such as comfort, security, decreased anxiety, and hope have been suggested. These alternates make us aware that caring is a nursing phenomenon, not a patient phenomenon. Others would counter that it evokes a patient-based response not possible in its absence. How might that patient response be labeled? Should the chief values in a theory rest in the nurse or in the patient?

REFERENCES

Boyd, C. O., & Munhall, P. (1989, November). A qualitative investigation of reassurance. *Holistic Nursing Practice, 1,* 61–69.

Ellis, R. (1969, July). The practitioner as theorist. *American Journal of Nursing, 7,* 1434–1438.

Gaut, D. A. (1986, July). Evaluating caring competencies in nursing practice. *Topics in Clinical Nursing, 2,* 77–83.

Geissler, E. M. (1991, April). Transcultural nursing and nursing diagnoses. *Nursing & Health Care, 4,* 190–192, 203.

Hutchinson, C. P., & Bahr, R. T. (1991, Summer). Types and meanings of caring behaviors among elderly nursing home residents. *Image, 2,* 85–88.

King, I. (1981). *A theory for nursing: Systems, concepts, process.* New York: Wiley.

Kreuter, F. R. (1957, May). What is good nursing care? *Nursing Outlook, 5,* 302–304.

Leininger, M. (1991). The theory of culture care diversity and universality. In M. Leininger, (Ed.), *Culture care diversity & universality: A theory of nursing* (pp. 5–68). New York: National League for Nursing Press.

Morse, J. M. (1992). Comfort: The refocusing of nursing care. *Clinical Nursing Research, 1,* 91–106.

Morse, J. M. (1996). The science of comforting. *Reflections, 4,* 6–8.

Morse, J. M., Bottorff, J., Neander, W., & Solberg, S. (1991, Summer). Comparative analysis of conceptualizations and theories of caring. *Image, 2,* 119–126.

Orem, D. E. (1985). *Nursing: Concepts of practice* (3rd ed). New York: McGraw-Hill.

Rawnsley, M. M. (1980, April). Toward a conceptual base for affective nursing. *Nursing Outlook, 4,* 244–250.

Roberts, J. E. (1990, March/April). Uncovering hidden caring. *Nursing Outlook, 2,* 67–69.

Styles, M. M. (1982). *On nursing: Toward a new endowment.* St. Louis: Mosby.

Swanson, K. M. (1991, May/June). Empirical development of a middle range theory of caring. *Nursing Research, 3,* 161–166.

Watson, J. (1979). *Nursing: The philosophy and science of caring.* Boston: Little, Brown.

Watson, J. (1988). *Nursing: Human science and human care: A theory of nursing.* New York: National League for Nursing Press.

Wiedenbach, E. (1963, November). The helping art of nursing. *American Journal of Nursing, 11,* 54–57.

Wiedenbach, E. (1970, May). Nurses' wisdom in nursing theory. *American Journal of Nursing, 5,* 1057–1062.

Wilber, K. (1979). *No boundary.* Los Angeles: Center Publications.

Wilber, K. (1980). *The Atman project: A transpersonal view of human development.* Wheaton, IL: Theosophical Publishing House.

Wolf, Z. R. (1986, July). The caring concept and nurse identified caring behaviors. *Topics in Clinical Nursing, 2,* 84–93.

7 Nursing: An Alternate Cure Ideology

For many theorists, care, as opposed to cure, was the historical factor differentiating nursing from medicine. Still today, theories that make caring the crux of nursing are strongly supported by many nurses. Yet cure is no longer the private territory of medicine; it is now claimed as legitimate turf for nursing activities, in regular nursing functions as well as in the work of nurse practitioners. We will look at the growth of cure theories in nursing after first looking at one nurse who radically opposed cure as nursing work.

CURE: NOT FOR NURSES, PLEASE

Lydia Hall (1968), anxious to differentiate between nursing and medicine, was convinced that cure belonged to medicine, not nursing. She was equally certain (in the 1960s) that cure was not possible in chronic care, which happened to be the specialty of her institution as well as an arena of care then assuming major importance. In this sense, one could say that Hall's theory was a theory of rehabilitation nursing and one of the first specialty theories to be developed. Of course, Hall did not see it that way at the time; she felt that she was writing for all of nursing.

By differentiating care and cure, Hall carved out a large territory for nursing—all of chronic care. She envisioned chronic care as a nursing domain, one where nurses would make the decisions, hiring physicians as needed for episodic cure needs. More importantly, she was able to bring off this vision in her facility.

Today, it seems ironic that anyone would use care, rather than cure, as the path to independent function, but that is exactly what Hall did. She used the care–cure dichotomy to carve out an independent domain of practice for nursing in an era when most of nursing was seen as dependent. The arguments that Hall (1968) used to differentiate care and care were interesting:

> *Nurses and others who work there (in hospitals) have got caught up in the CURE activities which are emphasized to the neglect of CARE, the kind that is essential in helping the patient get to the CORE of his difficulties through learning. (p. 2)*
>
> *When I ask physicians why they have not opened schools for practical doctors, as nurses faced with a shortage opened schools for practical nurses, I get an academic answer to an academic question. The truth is that physicians have not needed to open schools and will not, so long as they have "professional nurses" to whom they can delegate more and more medical tasks and activities. We have become "practical doctors" and so we say to the public by our behavior that we prefer being potential painers and practical doctors to being comforters and nurturers. (p. 1)*

Hall, a vehement protestor against nursing assuming cure-related activities, saw a patient has having three parts: (1) body, (2) pathology and treatment, and (3) person. Medicine, she claimed took care of pathology, and other professions such as the clergy lay claim to person, so nursing had the domain of the body. She insisted that the nurse be a caretaker and nurturer, not a "painer."

Ironically, as her theory evolves, the nurse only uses her access to the patient's body as a vehicle, and her real role is to help the patient get to the *core* of his problem. The core turns out to be the existential angst created by his chronic illness. The nurse helps the patient get to the core by techniques like mirroring (reflecting back his thoughts) and other psychological tactics. Her ultimate aim: whatever his physical abilities, that the patient develop a sense of self-mastery. Hall's three principles, care, cure, and core, which should have corresponded, respectively, to body, pathology, and person, got confused when the nurse, like the clergy, got into "core" (ie, person) work. Perhaps the remarkable part of this somewhat flawed theory is that Hall's nurses did make decisions in her facility; physicians were hired when a patient had a temporary illness requiring cure.

CURE: THE LIFE-REGULATING THEORIES

Loomis and Wood (1983, p. 7) also considered the nurse's role in chronic care, but the era had changed; the nurse's position had shifted on the spectrum of care versus cure. These authors took the position that the nurse is engaged in curing activities in just the same way that the physician is. Successful management of a chronic health deviation, they said, is the equivalent of cure, and that is within the legitimate realm of nursing practice.

Loomis and Wood agreed with Hall that chronic health care was the domain of nursing, yet they drew different conclusions about the nurse's role. Hall contended that the nurse must avoid cure activities; Loomis and Wood believed that what the nurse does *is* cure.

Patient teaching can be viewed as cure in many circumstances. Teaching the diabetic to regulate his own metabolism, as Loomis and Wood would assert, cures him to the extent that a chronic disease is curable, that is, to the extent that the condition is amenable to ongoing regulation. It is difficult to maintain that teaching the regulation of insulin, diet, and exercise is primarily a function of caring (affective).

In chronic care, admitting that nurses do cure work is simply a new perspective on an old role. Today, many traditional and new life-regulating strategies are used by nurses for patients. Stress management or smoking cessation programs might qualify. Nurses working with patients with acquired immunodeficiency syndrome (AIDS) could qualify on the Loomis and Wood model. For example, at the Columbia University School of Nursing, Dr. Anastasi is improving the quality of life for AIDS patients by helping them control severe diarrhea problems. Helping patients gain control of life-style problems such as drugs or alcohol abuse could also be perceived as curative under the Loomis and Wood model.

CURE: SUBORDINATING IT TO CARING

Sometimes theorists get around the care–cure dilemma by what some might call word games. For example, Watson (1979) *appears* to make the traditional differentiation between care and cure in deriving her so-called carative factors:

> *The term carative is used to contrast to the more common term curative to help the student to differentiate nursing and medicine. (p. 7)*

On further inspection, however, one sees that she has shifted the traditional meanings of care and cure:

> *Whereas curative factors aim at curing the patient of disease, carative factors aim at the caring process that helps the person attain (or maintain) health or die a peaceful death. (p. 7)*

In this formulation, Watson associates curing with disease in its narrowest meaning. Caring, on the other hand, is associated with healing the person. In that way, while eschewing *curing* for nurses, she brings them into the activity of healing. In effect, this brings nursing into the commonsense notion of curing, or, one might say, makes *curing* a limited aspect of a larger concept, *healing*. Caring, as Watson says, is more "healthogenic" than is curing (1979, p. 9).

In at least one book, Watson (1988a) advocates synthesizing care and cure. As she states, ". . . care is not proposed as simply a second-ary fall-back position when cure is impossible. Caring becomes the ethical principle or standard by which (curing) interventions are measured" (p. 2). In this change of tactics, she subordinates cure to care.

Leininger (1991) also subordinates cure to care when she says, "Care (caring) is essential to curing and healing, for there can be no curing without caring" (p. 45). Watson and Leininger both expand nursing's domain while decreasing medicine's, sometimes by manip-ulating the meaning of the terms, caring and curing (Watson, 1979), sometimes by asserting the dominance of care over cure (Leininger, 1991; Watson, 1988a).

CURE: SUBORDINATING IT TO HEALING

As Watson did in her later work, many theorists make a difference between curing and healing. McGlone (1990) notes that a disease is cured, whereas a person is healed. For McGlone healing means to be made whole, an awakening of a deeper sense of self (p. 78). Quinn (1989) describes healing as the realm of the nurse, whom she sees, not so much as healer but as midwife to an internal process in the patient:

> *Healing is a total, organismic, synergistic response that must emerge from within the individual if recovery and growth are to be accom-plished. . . . The Haelan Effect is the activation of the innate, diverse, synergistic, and multidimensional self-healing mechanism which mani-fests as emergence and repatterning of relationship. (p. 554)*

Often the theories that emphasize healing arise under the emerg-ing new world paradigm. One may get a quick flavor of this context in the following quotations from Watson:

> *A person's body is confined in time and space, but the mind and soul are not confined to the physical universe. One's higher sense of mind and soul transcends time and space and helps to account for notions like collective unconscious, causal past, mystical experiences, parapsy-chological phenomena, a higher sense of power, and may be an indicator of the spiritual evolution of human beings. (1988b, p. 50)*
> *The concept of the soul, as used here refers to the geist, spirit, inner self, or essence of the person, which is tied to a greater sense of self-*

awareness, a higher degree of consciousness, an inner strength, and a power that can expand human capacities and allow a person to transcend his or her usual self. The higher sense of consciousness and valuing of inner-self can cultivate a fuller access to the intuitive and even sometimes allow uncanny, mystical, or miraculous experiences. . . .

One's ability to transcend space and time occurs in a similar manner through one's mind, imagination, and emotions. Our bodies may be physically present in a given location or situation, but our minds and related feelings may be located elsewhere. (1988b, p. 46)

By characterizing her world in this way, Watson chooses a New Age ideology and alternate healing modalities. Watson's nurse enters "cure" work because cure—now healing—is no longer associated with the body, but with the individual's evolving personhood. The perception of disease has changed; as Watson says, it results from disharmony in the person. If nurses are instrumental in restoring harmony, they are involved in cure work.

The term *curing* is more often associated with the traditional medical model (and its related world view), whereas the term *healing* is typically associated with the emerging paradigm. Although there is crossover in use of these terms, curing and healing tend to evoke different images. Although Watson often uses the term curing, her connotations frequently evoke the notion of healing instead.

In nursing at the present, there are two different notions of healing. One is typified by Watson, in which an ordinary nurse–patient interpersonal relationship is seen as having healing potential. In Watson's terms, the process might help the patient establish harmony among body, mind, and spirit; and any good nurse might achieve this outcome. The second form of healing is closer to Quinn's (1996) use of New Age methods, especially therapeutic touch, restoring the patient's aura and making available to him a form of universal energy.

Therapeutic touch was first proposed in nursing by Krieger (1979, 1981), who borrowed the concept from nonnursing healers, where it has been used for centuries. This second form of healing, namely, the manipulation of forces and elements of man and the universe, requires special education not provided in all nursing education. Work with these energies, perceived and recognized as real by some but not all persons, is not unique to nursing. Indeed, there is a whole healing community comprised of all sorts of lay and health professions people, including many nurse members.

NONNURSING HEALING MOVEMENTS

The notion of healing is not the sole property of nursing, even though many nurses have laid claim to it. Just two of many such healing groups, each with their own related but discrete ideologies, are given here as illustration. The Barbara Brennan (1987, 1993) School of Healing is typical in the kind of world (context) it describes.

> *There is abundant evidence that many human beings today are expanding the usual five senses into super-sensory levels. Most people have High Sense Perception to some degree, without necessarily realizing it. . . . It is possible that there is already a transformation in consciousness taking place and that more people are developing a new sense in which information is received on different and possibly higher frequency. (1987, pp. 9–10)*

Brennan, not a nurse, holds a graduate degree in physics. She describes a "dynamic web of inseparable energy patterns," a notion of holistic awareness. She asserts that, "Holistic awareness will be outside linear time and three-dimensional space and therefore will not be easily recognized. We must practice holistic experience to be able to recognize it" (1987, p. 26).

Her school appears to be more rigorous than many other programs. Brennan's students are taught to use High Sense Perception of their patients' conditions for healing. For visualizers, this may include seeing the patients' auras and chakras (described as perceptible to those who have developed the ability to see at higher levels of vibration). Other students may have High Sense Perception through other senses, for example, touch.

Brennan's context is one in which multiple worlds exist in the same space, vibrating at different levels, making them, not unlike radio waves, undetectable except to those who can alter their vibratory rates of perception. Brennan's students use their hands to work in these altered frequencies, manipulating energy—pushing, pulling, or stopping it—to produce healing.

Brennan's healing program has some built-in controls. Her students are required to be in personal therapy, and the program attempts to validate the High Sense Perception of students. A major focus of the program is clarifying one's reception. Interpreting perceptions from higher vibrational levels *accurately*, happens as a matter of both training and personal growth and development. These elements comprise a major part of Brennan's theory as well as her program.

Brennan's healing philosophy handles flaws of body and psyche with the same therapies, treating the person holistically. Further, the healing therapies often are used simultaneously with modern medicine. Because they treat different phenomena (energy bodies and enfleshed bodies, respectively), there is no perceived conflict, even though both modalities share the goal of healing. The inherent interplay of body and psyche in Brennan's theory reminds one of Watson's assertion that disease arises from disharmony.

Reiki is another healing method that involves the movement of universal energies. Unlike the Brennan version, Reiki masters typically claim that the practitioner need not have something like High Sense Perception, that one can move the energies even in the absence of any perception of them. Where the Brennan school prepares its students to move energy through what appears to be creation of an altered state, that is, using meditation techniques to produce centering, grounding, and intentionality, the Reiki school has less focus on these elements when teaching the student to be a conduit for the energy. In the program, focus is placed on the practitioner having his four highest chakras open. Nor does the Reiki practitioner work with pushing and pulling the energy. The energy is simply transmitted to the patient and assumed to be "intelligent energy" that will go where it is needed. Because Reiki is practiced throughout this country and others, there is less uniformity in its teaching than in the Brennan school, and these comments may be skewed by the particular Reiki programs that I have witnessed.

Just as nursing seems to have borrowed the techniques of energy movement in its therapeutic touch, so the ministry uses similar powers in laying on of hands. MacNutt (1977) offers an example. Indeed, this religious usage may be one of the earliest forms of energy manipulation. The nurse does not have a corner in the "healing" market, despite much professional interest in the process.

A final word about the notion of therapeutic touch. The use of touch in the typical nursing model and the Brennan model are far apart, namely in the degree of skill required and the level of personal development needed by the healer. Krieger (1981), although admitting that there are levels of expertise in therapeutic touch, claims, ". . . basically, Therapeutic Touch is an act which nurses engage in quite naturally in the course of their nursing practice" (p. 138). In other words, on a primitive level, therapeutic touch is an instinctive act.

Therapeutic touch, as promulgated in nursing, sometimes is mistakenly conveyed more as a psychomotor skill, a technique for moving the hands over the patient's body in certain ways. The technique is sometimes being taught to nurses in a few days or a few hours in a concentrated workshop. Sometimes the teaching is superficial, with nurses given simple explanations of centering, grounding, and intention, without adequate time to acquire the altered levels of consciousness and meditative states required for achieving these elements of the process. One suspects that many nurses may think that they are delivering therapeutic touch when they are not.

Keegan (1995) describes the phases of therapeutic touch as follows:

1. *Centering oneself physically and psychologically; this is finding within oneself an inner reference of stability.*
2. *Exercising the natural sensitivity of the hand to assess the energy field of the client for clues to differentiate the quality of energy flow*
3. *Mobilizing areas in the client's energy field that the healer may perceive as being nonflowing (ie, sluggish, congested, or static)*
4. *Directing one's excess body energies to assist the client to repattern his or her own energies (p. 548)*

Seldom do therapeutic touch programs refer to the nature of the healer herself. As Heidt (1990) says, ". . . the nurse's field of energy may be characterized as being 'well' or 'whole'; the patient's energy field, as 'less whole'" (p. 180). I would call this an untested assumption. In contrast to the typical nursing model (that generally assumes all nurses qualify and can learn easily), Brennan has a 4-year program in which the healer's personal growth and her skills in directing energy are simultaneously developed and verified.

Do nurse teachers of therapeutic touch require any sort of High Sense Perception on the part of those learning the skill? Do they have methods of validating the student's skill? Programs with such safeguards are exceptions. The only validation in many nursing programs involves the confirmation by the student that she "feels" the energy. Others believe even this to be nonessential. For example, Quinn (1996) says that developing sensory perception of the patient's status comes with time, but that its absence does not impair the effectiveness of therapeutic touch. In this respect, she agrees with the Reiki position. Seldom is there any attempt to see if the student and instructor "feel" the same thing.

The issues here are multiple:

1. Whether such energy exists
2. Whether, if it exists, it can be manipulated and transmitted from one person to another
3. Whether the act of touch can be systematically effective in transmitting the energy apart from extensive training with verification
4. Whether or not the healer must herself have attained certain levels of personal development and requisite states of mind in which to exercise the skill

The rapid growth of healing programs is one of the more interesting facets of the so-called New Age world view. Although nurses have been heavily involved in healing therapies, the territory of healing is not likely to ever be exclusive to the nursing profession. In the first place, many of the most successful healers are not nurses, and the therapies associated with healing are not taught in most nursing programs.

Many of the nurses who move into healing work come from programs like Watson's, curricula that stress holistic theories, often those more or less linked to Roger's theory. Although not all holistic theories embrace healing, many have a context not unlike that proposed by Watson or Brennan.

The holistic nursing movement (in many of its formulations) grants that nurses may be agents of cure, with therapies such as therapeutic touch. Unlike the cure theories advanced by Loomis and Wood, unlike the cure work of nurse practitioners, holistic theories typically offer cure work that little resembles the cure work of physicians. Cure is the goal, but the therapies are radically different. Almost invariably, these theories are grounded in an alternate world paradigm. Nor do all practitioners assert that therapeutic touch cures; many focus on its ability to produce relaxation and relieve stress and pain.

SUMMARY

The issue of care versus cure is more complex than it might appear at first glance. Can health care actions be truly segregated on this basis? Is every act of a health care worker aimed specifically at either care or cure? Can the same act serve both goals? Can the same act serve one goal at one time and its opposite at another?

Must the content of medicine and nursing remain inviolable? Border setting between nursing and medicine may be seen as a political position rather than an eternal truth. The difference may be what we chose to make it in our particular nation at a particular time in history. One might contrast the United States system with that in the various Soviet countries, where the nursing role is structured as an interim rung on the way to the medicine role. In that system, the two professions are not differentiated in kind but are on a continuum. Our practitioner movement may be taking us in that direction.

Caring and curing are perennial goals in health care. At present, numerous movements account for both of these goals within the scope of nursing practice. Nevertheless, a large number of nurses and nurse theorists still use care versus cure as the demarcation between the professions of nursing and medicine. Nor is it possible to say out of context, what either term (caring or curing) means. Nursing theorists have given both terms many and varied connotations and denotations.

REFERENCES

Brennan, B. A. (1987). *Hands of light: A guide to healing through the human energy field.* New York: Bantam Books.

Brennan, B. A. (1993). *Light emerging: The journey of personal healing.* New York: Bantam Books.

Hall, L. (1968, Spring). Another view of nursing care and quality. *Maryland Nursing News, 1,* 1–5.

Heidt, P. R. (1990, Fall). Openness: A qualitative analysis of nurses' and patients' experiences of therapeutic touch. *Image, 3,* 180–186.

Keegan, L. (1995). Touch: Connecting with the healing power. In B. M. Dossey, L. Keegan, C. E. Guzetta, & L. G. Kolkmeier (Eds.), *Holistic health promotion: A guide for practice* (2nd ed., pp. 539–569). Rockville, MD: Aspen.

Krieger, D. (1979). *The therapeutic touch: How to use your hands to help or to heal.* Englewood Cliffs, NJ: Prentice-Hall.

Krieger, D. (1981). *Foundations for holistic health nursing practices: The Renaissance nurse.* Philadelphia: Lippincott.

Leininger, M. M. (1991). The theory of culture care diversity and universality. In M. M. Leininger (Ed.), *Culture care diversity & universality: A theory of nursing* (pp. 5–68). New York: National League for Nursing.

Loomis, M. E., & Wood, D. J. (1983, Winter). Cure: The potential outcome of nursing care. *Image, 1,* 4–7.

MacNutt, F. (1977). *The power to heal.* Notre Dame, IN: Ave Maria Press.

McGlone, M. E. (1990, July). Healing the spirit. *Holistic Nursing Practice, 4,* 77–84.

Quinn, J. (1996). *Therapeutic touch: A home study course for family caregivers: Everyone a healer.* [Videotape]. New York: National League for Nursing.

Quinn, J. F. (1989, December). On healing, wholeness, and the Haelan effect. *Nursing & Health Care, 10,* 552–556.

Watson, J. (1979). *Nursing: The philosophy and science of caring,* Boston: Little, Brown.

Watson, J. (1988a). Introduction: An ethic of caring/curing/nursing *qua* nursing. In J. Watson & M. A. Ray (Eds.), *The ethics of care and the ethics of cure: Synthesis in chronicity* (pp. 1–3). New York: National League for Nursing Press.

Watson, J. (1988b). *Nursing: Human science and human care.* New York: National League for Nursing Press.

8 *Holistic Nursing Theories*

Holistic theories represent the fastest growing trend in nursing. A *holistic theory* is one whose subject matter is conceptualized as an indivisible whole, an entity that is fractured and distorted if considered as a collection of parts. Most often the subject matter of holistic theories is man, but some holistic theories take the universe or health as subject matter. Whatever their subject matter, holistic theories share a commitment not to see their subject matter as an accumulation of parts. They take a view counter to the predominant medical model as well as to many popular nursing models.

THE INFLUENCE OF ROGERS

Martha Rogers (1970, 1990, 1994) was one of the earlier nurse theorists to promulgate a holistic theory. Indeed, many subsequent holistic theories have adopted her notions of man and environment. As she says:

> *The unity of man is a reality. Man interacts with his environment in his totality. Only as man's wholeness is perceived does the study of man begin to yield meaningful concepts and theories. Only as man's oneness is apprehended is it possible to identify man's distinctive attributes. (1970, p. 44)*
> *Nursing is the study of unitary, irreducible, indivisible human and environmental fields: people and their world. (1990, p. 6)*
> *. . . people are energy fields. They do not have them. All reality is postulated to be multidimensional as defined herein. One does not become multidimensional. Rather, this is a way of perceiving reality. (1990, pp. 5–6)*

Rogers's original theory focused around principles of (1) reciprocy (interaction between human and environmental fields), (2) synchrony (a function of the human/environmental field interacting at a point in space-time), (3) helicy (subsuming reciprocy and synchrony and describing the unidirectional life process as characterized by probablistic goal-directedness), and (4) resonancy (purporting that change in pattern and organization of the human and environmental field is propagated in waves) (Rogers, 1970, pp. 95–103).

Her newer version has reduced those principles to three:

- *Principle of Resonancy: continuous change from lower to higher frequency wave patterns in human and environmental fields*
- *Principle of Helicy: continuous innovative, unpredictable, increasing diversity of human and environmental field patterns*
- *Principle of Integrality: continuous mutual human field and environmental field process (Rogers, 1990, p. 8)*

Although these principles may seem complex, especially because Rogers creates her own vocabulary, a close examination reveals a world paradigm not unlike that of Watson and Brennan.

THEORISTS IN THE ROGERIAN TRADITION

Newman, Parse, Fitzpatrick, and many other holistic nurse theorists credit Rogers with having been the inspiration for their work. Roger's (1970) early book, known as the Purple Book by her students, primarily portrayed a view of the world and man (context). There was much room for students to take her world view and expand on it or to evolve specifics of nursing therapy compatible with her view.

Take, for example, the work of Black and Haight (1992, pp. 8–9) who applied Roger's principle of integrality to late life development. They looked at the final phase of life review through the principle of integrality and differentiated between mere reminiscing and an integrality that included evaluating and garnering insight from the life experience.

Today many nurses with holistic theories believe they are doing "the same thing" because of their mutual beginnings in Roger's work. Consider the theories of Newman (1979, 1986, 1994), Parse (1981), and Krieger (1979, 1981); it is clear that each has added unique components and taken slightly different directions.

Sometimes the difference among holistic theories is one of focus rather then substance. For example, some of these theories look more closely at health than at man, and some take the opposite course. The reader may get a taste of holistic theory differences and similarities from the representative citations given here.

Newman virtually joins the subjects of health and man by saying that the natural evolution of man *is* health. For Newman (1994), health is equated with the evolution of consciousness. Like Watson, she follows closely the models of psychology cited in the transpersonal literature.

> *The process of the evolution of consciousness is the process of health. The human being comes from a state of potential consciousness into the world of determinate matter and have the capacity for understanding that enables them to gain insight regarding their patterns. This instantaneous insight represents a turning point in evolving consciousness with concomitant gains in freedom of action. (p. 43)*
>   *. . . the "flow of life" seen as a kaleidoscopic evolution of patterning with paradoxes, contradictions, and ambiguities continually being synthesized into insights that lead to an ever-expanding consciousness. The revolutional conceptualization of Newman's paradigm is the proposition that health is the synthesis of disease/nondisease. Newman's model embraces a dialectic outlook where transformation is basic, where the fundamental unit of analysis is movement, and where disease and nondisease are each reflections of a larger whole. (1986, p. 111)*

The focus on patterning is reminiscent of Rogers's early work, where she says such things as: "Pattern and organization have become basic concepts in contemporary efforts to achieve a better understanding of human growth and behavior" (1970, p. 61). Or, "The life process possesses its own dynamic pattern and organization. The patterning that takes place over time is evolutionary in nature and encompasses the unity of life" (1970, p. 62).

Newman (1986) also adopts Rogers's notion of energy fields:

> *Although we cannot always "see" energy exchange, we accept that it is a characteristic of the human field (eg, the energy patterns depicted by an electrocardiogram or electroencephalogram). Disease makes it possible for us to envision a total pattern of the energy field of a person. For example, hypertension may connote a pattern of contained energy, hyperthyroidism a pattern of diffuse, multidirectional energy, or diabetes the inability to use available energy. (pp. 22–23)*

Krieger (1981), following Roger's work, takes a holistic perspective of health in which man and environment are both essential components:

> *The underlying premise of holistic health practices is that it is a major misconception of our times that the germ theory accounts for all illness. . . . This means that illness is the product of a complementary interaction between mind and body under conditions of stress that cannot be reconciled. The goal of the holistic perspective is to treat all aspects of*

the person's problems by an integrated approach that considers both the person in the context of the problem and the problem in the context of the uniqueness of the individual, thus giving the situation a more humanistic orientation than has previously been the case. (pp. 79–80)

Parse (1981), like Rogers, develops her own vocabulary of preferred terms. Here, she discusses what she calls the coconstituting of man and environment:

Assumption 1 synthesized the concepts of coexistence, coconstitution, and pattern and organization. The assumption means that man exists with others, evolving simultaneously and in cadence with the environment. Man, a recognizable pattern in the man-environment interrelationship, unfolds with contemporaries the ideas of predecessors. This interrelationship is the continuity that connects past with future, bearing witness to man's coexistence with all men. (p. 26)

Man and environment interchange energy to create what is in the world, and man chooses the meaning given to the situations he cocreates. Man is responsible for all outcomes of choices even though he does not know them when making a decision. (p. 27)

Most holistic theories in nursing take a transcendental view of man or reality, that is, they perceive the most real facets of existence to be principles and experiences that reach beyond the concrete, measurable, everyday experience. They share a general displeasure with any reductionist thinking, that is, with any theory that explains a thing by reference to its parts.

NON-ROGERIAN HOLISM

Not all holistic theories give evidence of being direct spin-offs from Rogers. Kolcaba (1992), for example, devises a map for holistic comfort that would be compatible with a more traditional world view, yet still preserves the holism. Her model is designed to create, as she says, a nurse-sensitive outcome (p. 1). In her grid, she interfaces two sets of variables in order that comfort be seen as a multidimensional, personal experience, with different degrees of intensity. Her cognitive map looks at physical, psychospiritual, environmental, and social factors as they cross-grid against states of relief, ease, or transcendence.

Selder (1989) also develops a holistic theory that is neither derived from nor representative of Rogers's unitary man paradigm. Hers is a theory of life transition, described as follows:

A life transition is initiated when a person's current reality is disrupted. The disruption of the reality can originate in a crucial event or from a determined decision. (p. 437)

Life transition theory describes how people restructure their reality and resolve uncertainty, a major characteristic of any transition. The shape of the transition is the resolution of the uncertainty. (p. 437)

Selder's theory, though it retains an holistic approach to man, focuses on the unique perceptions of the person undergoing transition. For example, she says in relation to the perception of time (one of the elements altered by transition):

During the life transition there are changes in the perception of time. Following a disruption in reality, the person's sense of time is collapsed; there is no orientation to the future as far as time is concerned, there is preoccupation with the predisrupted reality. (p. 451)

Selder's model is middle range, that is, not purporting to apply to all persons or even all persons labeled as patients. It applies to a single class: those who have experienced a major life disruption. Her work involves, for example, patients suffering spinal cord injuries.

Fitzpatrick (1983) also is concerned with temporal patterns, but extends her theory to all mankind:

This life perspective rhythm model . . . proposes that the process of human development is characterized by rhythms. . . . Throughout the developmental process one can identify peaks and troughs of particular human rhythms with the overall progression toward faster rhythms. For example, in relation to temporal patterns one can identify the basic progression of the rhythm as moving from time passing slowly, through time passing quickly, toward timelessness. (p. 300)

The theories of Selder and Fitzpatrick could be compatible if filtered through the same world view; yet the Selder theory could have validity in a more traditional world view as well. Not all holistic theories have to view the world through the same paradigm. The fact that many holistic theories come out of Rogerian notions or New Age ideology is chance, not necessity. Some theories, like Selder's, might apply in more than one world construct.

HOLISTIC THEORIES: WEAKNESSES AND STRENGTHS

Man in his totality is the subject matter for most holistic theories of nursing. Some theorists, like Newman, have equated health with human development; others like Watson, see health as a form of human harmony. Holistic theories face a boundary problem when it comes to nursing, and we could rightly ask: How does the nurse differ from the transpersonal psychologist? Often these theories are dense with world context, heavy on how man is seen in his environment, and thin on what nurses actually do. In other cases, a strange dichotomy exists between what nurses do in their actual practice and the topics that the theories discuss.

Another issue related to these theories can be framed in this way: If nursing is the study of man in his totality, how does that relate to the fact that the average man thinks of a nurse as someone who helps when his health fails. If many of these holistic theories are to be taken literally, there is no more justification for a nurse when someone is ill than when the person is well. It seems that everyone needs a nurse (someone to assist in human development) apart from considerations of wellness or illness. If that is so, how can a person be convinced that the nurse has all the knowledge and skill necessary to be that lifetime guide?

In taking an holistic image of man as its subject matter, nursing is able to contrast its subject matter (whole man) with medicine's (man as his physiologic body systems, man as a collection of diseases). The assertion of holistic nursing theories is that medicine treats the disease, whereas nursing treats the person. This is not to say that physicians would agree with this interpretation.

THE QUESTION OF METHOD IN HOLISM

Another issue raised by holistic theories is how one studies, researches, or practices with a whole that cannot be divided. Some theorists get around this problem by having the nurse "intuit" the patient, somewhat akin to the old philosophical argument given by Gibson (1960) in relation to social inquiry:

> *The central notion, as we have seen, is that we understand what is going on simply by participating in it. This is easily recognized in the case of ourselves; we live through our own experiences, and in doing so become aware of them. But we also participate, along with others, in social processes, and in doing this are able to grasp the situation not only from our own point of view, but from theirs. By identifying ourselves with them, we come to feel what they feel, or at any rate to think their thoughts. (p. 50)*

Others have no problem separating out aspects of the whole on a temporary, provisional basis. Krieger (1981) describes the mechanism this way:

> *In terms of humans, the plan of the whole means that practices to support a person's health must keep the self-identity of the "whole" person in mind and must recognize that it is from this enduring perspective that each individual perceives intrinsic reality. This intrinsic reality, based as it is upon the individual's life history, in turn lends the individ-*

ual personality a unity of character for its expression. Consequently, the emerging stance of the holistic health practitioner is to strive to understand simultaneously the relationship of the "part" of the individual under concern to the totality of that individual's interactions and the relationship of the whole to its parts. (p. 4)

Moccia (1986) also addresses the issue of how one considers parts in a holistic theory:

Once holism is assumed, one must find a way to recognize, acknowledge, respect and account for the inevitable distortions that occur when the indivisible totality is artificially divided, as is necessary. Such a process is described within a dialectical understanding of reality by the act of individuation, which is "simply a matter of carving up the whole in a different manner for a particular purpose." I have argued elsewhere that this concept offers nursing scholarship a way out of the theoretical paradox that comes with holism. (p. 31)

Newman (1986) may be on thinner ice when she accepts use of a tool specifically associated with a reductionist theory:

In spite of this belief that pattern recognition is more a matter of being able to "read" one's own pattern than of collecting information "external" to oneself, an assessment framework may be useful in initial efforts to identify pattern. The assessment framework developed by the nurse theorist group of the North American Nursing Diagnosis Association (NANDA) is consistent with the paradigm of health presented here. (p. 73)

Although one may quibble concerning which methods have infringed too sharply on the indivisible whole, it is clear that one can look at the same subject matter through various colored glasses (ie, partialities) as a method of individuating while yet preserving the whole. For Levine's theory, one might look at the whole patient through energy-colored glasses at one time and structure-colored glasses at another without destroying the integrity and unity of the whole human being.

Holistic theories have both a philosophical commitment not to see things in a reductionist fashion and an obligation to find appropriate practice/research/learning methods. Because the classical experimental design, with its manipulation of variables, breaks things into component parts, it is difficult to combine it with holism. Holism has found more acceptable methods in phenomenology or hermeneutics. Both of these methods explore the lived experience as it is immediately experienced; both aim for a deeper understanding of the phenomenon observed, with hermeneutics focusing on the interpretation of such experience.

Because these methods lend themselves to more global subject matters, it is common to find holistic theorists interested in conditions of the human spirit—or the emotive aspects of experience that arise concurrently with illness. For example, Dugan (1989) analyzes sadness, fear, and anger, finding that these human conditions can, if prolonged and deep, develop into states of illnesses: depression, anxiety, and hostility/resentment, respectively.

Globally, one could say, theorists who are reductionists (focus on the parts) tend to use quantitative research and classical experimental design. Advocates of holistic theories, on the other hand, usually prefer qualitative research. Because the two philosophies represent different ways of viewing the world (in wholes, in parts), it is not surprising that they differ as to what sources will be taken as valid in searching for truth. Benner (1985) states the problem from the perspective of qualitative research:

> *The paradox of the subject/object split of Cartesian dualism is that it is either extremely subjectivizing or extremely objectifying. The self is viewed as a possession and attributes are given objectively as possessions by the subject in a purely intentional way. This view cannot take account of the historical, cultural, embodied, situated person. (p. 2)*

Some researchers simply cannot accept methods that fail to objectify and isolate variables. They insist that qualitative research cannot lead to knowledge. Researchers who favor qualitative research (and that includes most who adopt holistic theories) believe that much of what is significant is lost in the act of objectifying and isolating parts. Of course, not every researcher is for one method and against the other. Most nurses realize that each method has much to offer. However, phenomenology and hermeneutics fit well with holistic theory development because they allow for the study of a subject matter in its entirety, without artificially separating it into pieces.

One may look the reductionist and holistic methods of research, and find, as we will discuss in Chapter 20, that one approach represents inquiry into the sensate world (using measurement) and one represents inquiry into the world of mind (using intellectual apprehension). The argument presented in Chapter 20 is that these different worlds require different methods of knowing.

Holistic perceptions and those that break things into parts are sometimes confused when a partial view is comprehensive—meaning that it contains all its parts. Many theorists mistakenly claim to be holistic when what they actually mean is that they consider all the components. Considering all the pieces is *not* a holistic tactic. An holistic phenomenon has only one essence in which all aspects participate. The two notions of "wholeness" are antithetical ways of viewing man and the world.

As illustration, one could consider the nursing process. It can be applied in its totality to a patient, but that does not make it holistic. The nurse must divide things into steps and pieces in her mind, calling forth thought patterns that look at the parts. In contrast, the dialectic thought process, which strives to blend perceived entities into larger, more comprehensive wholes, allows for holism. Here, like in Newman, the human being might be considered a small hologram of, or an indivisible part of the larger world—in this case, the world of evolving consciousness. The latter approach is compatible with phenomenology, yet can be separated from it. Because most nurses are counseled to treat the whole patient, not the incision, not the broken leg, holistic philosophies appeal to many. Indeed, these theories are threatening to eclipse the nursing process theory in popularity.

HOLISTIC CURING

In the last chapter, we said that the holistic nursing movement often advocates the nurse as cure agent. Many practitioners of holistic nursing claim they have created viable cure alternatives to medical practice. Others claim they do curing work that is compatible with and complementary to medicine.

Holistic nurse practitioners often adopt independent nursing interventions that may be applied with a curing rather than a caring intention (or they may be applied as both anodyne and cure simultaneously). Therapeutic touch (Krieger, 1981, 1993; Quinn, 1988, 1996) was the first such method to gain extensive popularity in nursing, although it has been followed by others.

Therapeutic touch is not always separated from a religious or spiritual aspect, as we will see in the next chapter. Where the two aspects are conjoined, often the spiritual interpretation is closer to New Age beliefs than to older religious forms. As Krieger (1981) says about therapeutic touch:

> *Therapeutic Touch derives from, but is not the same as, the ancient art of the laying-on of hands. The major points of difference between Therapeutic Touch and the laying-on of hands are methodological; Therapeutic Touch has no religious base as does the laying-on-of hands; it is a conscious, intentional act; it is based on research findings; and Therapeutic Touch does not require a declaration of faith from the healee (patient) for it to be effective. (p. 138)*

Like Krieger, many nurses separate therapeutic touch and religion (which has a parallel in laying on of hands). Other parallels could be made between New Age therapies and religious practices; for example, one might compare meditation and centering to religious meditation.

Therapeutic touch has remained one of the chief methods used in holistic curing, but guided imagery, acupuncture, and other holistic techniques are also used. Barrett (1990) gives a generic description of methods that she sees developing under the holistic theory of Rogers. She raises the point that human contact may be an important part of the procedures:

> *Practice modalities are options that can be used by clients to pursue a way of living, to assist in lifestyle change, to increase awareness of opportunities to be well, and to provide information that may be helpful in making health-related choices.*
>
> *Many modalities can promote power enhancement whereby clients use their capacity to participate knowingly in change to actualize certain potentials. . . .*
>
> *At times the deliberative mutual patterning process itself is the healing modality. This is the case when human therapeutic contact is deemed essential to enhancing the health of the person. (p. 34)*

New holistic methods are numerous, and a wide armamentarium of techniques is developing rapidly. Hare (1988), for example, explores shiatsu acupressure, a method akin to acupuncture, and Titlebaum (1988) discusses relaxation therapy. Ruxton (1988) and Dugan (1989), following on Norman Cousins's (1979) lead, explore humor in its curative potential. Barnum (1989) discusses the lending of energy, and White (1988) expands on the use of the hands for therapeutic massage. Zahourek (1987) explores clinical hypnosis, and Brallier (1988) uses biofeedback. Dossey (1995a, 1995b, 1997) discuss cognitive therapy, imagery, and music therapy, among other methods.

Holistic theorists are among those who interpret nursing as mixing caring and curing. It is clear, for example, that Krieger's use of the term, healer, is not to be taken lightly. It is often difficult to categorize these methods as care or cure work. For example, Kist (1992) used acupuncture to keep pregnant drug abusers "clean" in the latter months of pregnancy. How could this successful therapy be classified as care or cure?

Vines (1988), Krieger (1981), and Dossey (1995a) all use guided imagery, possibly the second most popular technique after therapeutic touch. Dossey describes it this way:

> *The dramatic psychophysiologic changes that occur in imagery and hypnosis result from gaining access to state-dependent memory, learning, and behavior systems and making their encoded information available for problem solving. Every time the client gains access to such information, he or she has an opportunity to reframe experiences and develop new health behaviors/thoughts. (p. 612)*

Dossey (1995a) explains the effectiveness of imagery in the following way:

The conversion or transformation of information/energy from one form to another is transduction. The mind can be seen as nature's supreme way of receiving, generating, and transducing information. . . . New ideas and events evoke bodymind changes; that is, neural pathways and consciousness connect to permit information transduction. (p. 9)

Vines (1988, p. 36) concurs, noting that mental images are not pictures in the mind but notions that may be integrated with the individual's physiologic response patterns.

Guided imagery, like therapeutic touch, has been adopted by nurses more often than by physicians, although that is changing with time. Inroads have been made among physicians by new paradigm works such as those by Dr. Larry Dossey (1982), by funding now available to research new methods, and by recent changes in reimbursement for such therapies.

Holistic methods appeal to nurses who believe that humans respond on levels other than the merely physiologic. As B. Dossey (1996b) explained, however, such methods may have more of a physiologic base than is usually credited to them. Indeed, there is much new physiologic research just beginning to reach the literature about subtle inter-bodymind effects (as Dossey calls them). It may be that in the future many of the holistic therapeutics will become mainstream because of a shifting version of the human functioning, even within the scientific paradigm. In any case, holistic methods avoid the reductionism that is the crux of the holistic complaint against other nursing theories.

Holism, then, whether applied to the patient, to health, or to the whole of reality, is a commitment to seeing the subject matter as indivisible, not as a composition of smaller parts. Holism is not a method but a philosophy, a commitment to viewing its subject matter in its entirety. Its research is most compatible with a phenomenological approach (including derivatives such as hermeneutics or critical social approach). A dialectic thought process is often compatible with holism as well. Phenomenology and dialectic thought are discussed later in this book.

SUMMARY

Most holistic theories of nursing deal with content such as transpersonal psychology, aspects of transition and temporality, and concepts of self-growth as healing. These subjects must be analyzed carefully to evaluate whether or not they represent the appropriate domain for the profession of nursing or whether they more appropriately belong to minister or psychologist. Not every nurse will reach the same conclusion.

The holistic theories tend to be presented within a New Age

ideology, although some few are contained in or compatible with a traditional world view. Subject matters of these theories range from man, to health, to human evolution, to the universe itself. At present, holistic theories vie for predominance with those based on nursing process/nursing diagnosis. These two sorts of theories form a new professional dichotomy, one that holds little hope for resolution. Will the two philosophies, with their related methods, develop two radically different schools of nursing? Or will one side eventually become normative? The answer is yet to be determined.

REFERENCES

Barnum, B. J. (1989, November/December). Expanded consciousness: Nurses' experiences. *Nursing Outlook, 6*, 260–266.

Barrett, E. A. M. (1990). Rogers' science-based nursing practice. In E. A. M. Barrett (Ed.), *Visions of Rogers' science-based nursing* (pp. 31–44). New York: National League for Nursing Press.

Benner, P. (1985, October). Quality of life: A phenomenological perspective on explanation, prediction, and understanding in nursing science. *Advances in Nursing Science, 1*, 1–14.

Black, G., & Haight, B. K. (1992, October). Integrality as a holistic framework for the life-review process. *Holistic Nursing Practice, 1*, 7–15.

Brallier, L. W. (1988, May). Biofeedback and holism in clinical practice. *Holistic Nursing Practice, 3*, 26–33.

Cousins, N. (1979). *Anatomy of an illness*, New York: Norton.

Dossey, B. M. (1995a). Imagery: Awakening the inner healer. In B. M. Dossey, L. Keegan, C. E. Guzzetta, & L. G. Kolkmeier, *Holistic nursing: A handbook for practice* (2nd ed., pp. 609–666). Gaithersburg, MD: Aspen.

Dossey, B. M. (1995b). The psychophysiology of bodymind healing. In B. M. Dossey, L. Keegan, C. E., Guzzetta, & L. G. Kolkmeier, *Holistic nursing: A handbook for practice* (2nd ed., pp. 87–111). Gaithersburg, MD: Aspen.

Dossey, B. M. (Ed.). (1997). *Core curriculum for holistic nursing.* Gaithersburg, MD: Aspen.

Dossey, L. (1982). *Space, time & medicine.* Boston: New Science Library.

Dugan, D. O. (1989). Laughter and tears: Best medicine for stress. *Nursing Forum, 1*, 18–26.

Fitzpatrick, J. (1983). A life perspective rhythm model. In J. Fitzpatrick & A. Whall (Eds.), *Conceptual models of nursing: Analysis and application* (pp. 295–302). Bowie, MD: Robert J. Brady.

Gibson, Q. (1960). *The logic of social inquiry.* London: Routledge & Kegan Paul.

Hare, M. L. (1988, May). Shiatsu acupressure in nursing practice. *Holistic Nursing Practice, 3*, 68–74.

Kist, K. O. (1992, October 28). *The research role of the clinical nurse specialist as a marketing tool.* Paper presented at the Seventh Annual Clinical

Specialist Symposium, Hunter-Bellevue School of Nursing, City University of New York, New York.

Kolcaba, K. Y. (1992, September). Holistic comfort: Operationalizing the construct as a nurse-sensitive outcome. *Advances in Nursing Science, 1*, 1–10.

Krieger, D. (1979). *The therapeutic touch: How to use your hands to help or to heal.* Englewood Cliffs, NJ: Prentice-Hall.

Krieger, D. (1981). *Foundations for holistic health nursing practices: The Renaissance nurse.* Philadelphia: Lippincott.

Krieger, D. (1993). *Accepting your power to heal: A personal practice of therapeutic touch.* Santa Fe, NM: Bear & Company Publishing.

Moccia, P. (1986). Theory development and nursing practice: A synopsis of a study of the theory-practice dialect. In P. Moccia (Ed.), *New approaches to theory development* (pp. 23–38). New York: National League for Nursing Press.

Newman, M. (1979). *Theory development in nursing.* Philadelphia: Davis.

Newman, M. A. (1986). *Health as expanding consciousness.* St. Louis: Mosby.

Newman, M. (1994). *Health as expanding consciousness.* New York: National League for Nursing Press.

Parse, R. R. (1981). *Man-living-health: A theory of nursing.* New York: Wiley.

Quinn, J. (1988). Building a body of knowledge: Research on therapeutic touch. *Journal of Holistic Nursing, 1*, 37–45.

Quinn, J. (1996). *Therapeutic touch: A home study course for family caregivers: Everyone a healer.* [Videotape]. New York: National League for Nursing Press.

Rogers, M. E. (1970). *An introduction to the theoretical basis of nursing.* Philadelphia: Davis.

Rogers, M. E. (1990). Nursing: Science of unitary, irreducible, human beings: Update 1990. In E. A. M. Barrett (Ed.), *Visions of Rogers' science-based nursing* (pp. 5–11). New York: National League for Nursing Press.

Rogers, M. E. (1994). Nursing science evolves. In M. Madrid & E. A. M. Barrett (Eds.), *Rogers' scientific art of nursing practice* (pp. 3–9). New York: National League for Nursing Press.

Ruxton, J. P. (1988, May). Humor intervention deserves our attention. *Holistic Nursing Practice, 3*, 54–62.

Selder, F. (1989, October). Life transition theory: The resolution of uncertainty. *Nursing & Health Care, 8*, 437–451.

Titlebaum, H. M. (1988, May). Relaxation. *Holistic Nursing Practice, 3*, 17–25.

Vines, S. W. (1988, May). The therapeutics of guided imagery. *Holistic Nursing Practice, 3*, 34–44.

White, J. A. (1988, May). Touching with intent: Therapeutic massage. *Holistic Nursing Practice, 3*, 63–67.

Zahourek, R. P. (1987, November). Clinical hypnosis in holistic nursing. *Holistic Nursing Practice, 1*, 15–24.

9 *Spirituality and Ethics in Nursing Theory*

SPIRITUALITY AND ETHICS: THE SAME? DIFFERENT?

In an earlier chapter, we talked about the difference between healing and curing, noting that the terminology of healing was often applied in newer paradigms. Further, many theorists saw curing as only a small component of healing. Healing was applied to the person, curing to the disease. A similar situation applies to spirituality and ethics. Although both have to do with morality, with what is right and wrong, they connote different images, different ways of handling oneself in the world.

The term *ethics* is more in keeping with older theories and an older world view. It focuses on rights and duties, on equity and justice, often with a rule orientation. *Spirituality* is a term more often found in theories arising in New Age paradigms or in association with religions.

Although ethics calls forth an image of a code of acceptable behavior, spirituality calls forth an image of life lived and experienced in light of certain beliefs and sensitivities. As the terms have been used in nursing, the tendency is for discussions of *ethics* to be connected to problems or vulnerabilities—situations in which the nurse might do the wrong thing.

Spirituality, on the other hand, has been related to the joyous experiences of soul growth and connection with a higher good, however envisioned. We might call spirituality the larger term, ethics the more limited one. This is not to say that there is no crossover in the vocabulary in nursing theories.

Watson (1988) captures the difference in connotation in the following:

A nurse may perform actions toward a patient out of a sense of duty or moral obligation, and would be an ethical nurse. Yet it may be false to say he or she cared about the patient. The value of human care and caring involves a higher sense of spirit of self. (p. 31)

We begin our comparison and contrast of the two ideologies by looking at the renewed focus on the spiritual aspect of nursing.

SPIRITUAL ASPECTS OF NURSING

Despite nursing's strong historical roots in religion, it has been a long time since nurses (outside of religious schools and institutions) talked about the spiritual side of nursing. In eras past when nursing was striving to prove itself a science, even its language changed, deleting earlier references to spiritual values. As Donley (1991) said:

Doctors acted like scientists, businessmen, or entrepreneurs. Nurses were also co-opted by the glamour and power of high-technology nursing. As some of the art and most of the mystery of healing were lost, it became clear to nurses, and others who worked in hospitals, that they were part of a technical money-making system, not a "sacred system." (p. 178)

In the last two decades, older descriptions of nursing as caring for the mind, body, and spirit were replaced by references to biopsychosocial man. True, there were diseases of the body and mind, but seldom did anyone refer to diseases of the spirit. Few theories of nursing involved the idea of spirit as an essential component. Only a few schools of nursing (those affiliated with strict religious sects) retained courses on religion in their curricula or required church attendance. In these programs, religious values were included in the life of the students, but seldom entered directly into nursing theory formulation for patient care. At best, one could say that spirituality formed an assumed context, an understanding that the nurses in the organization would act out of these motives.

Longway (1970), writing for the *Journal of Adventist Education*, was one of the few theorists who made a religious notion central to her theory. Working within a framework of holism, she defined a circuit of wholeness in which man had unlimited potential for growth and development, a wholeness denoting harmony among parts (p. 21). To that notion she added the idea of God as the source of man's power—and it was power that could be cut off if a man fell out of the plan of redemption (pp. 21–22). Disease was a stoppage in man's power, and healing was the restoration of power by providing energy, which she described in this way:

> *The method whereby energy is made available to man is by giving, motivated by love, for giving completes the circuit of God, the source of power. (p. 22)*
>
> *The aim of intervention is to supply energy to the individual, help him to lay hold of more energy for himself and thus to enable him to advance along the illness-wellness continuum as far as his limitations will permit. (p. 22)*

This description comes close to some of the modern theories related to New Age paradigms. Because Longway's nurse heals by supplying energy, the theory is one in which the nurse is a healer as well as caretaker.

SPIRITUALITY IN NEWER NURSING THEORIES

Longway's theory was published over 20 years ago, but it did not start a spiritual resurgence. That had to wait until the emergence of a new world paradigm. Now nurses are looking at spirituality again and struggling to define the concept. Newman (1989) notes that holy, whole, and heal all come from the same root meaning (p. 1). Hover-Kramer (1989, p. 29) seeks to locate spirituality in the search for wholeness and the surrender to a reality greater than ourselves. Her position is much like that of transpersonal psychologists who see the spiritual as an emergent stage of growth.

Clark, Cross, Deane, and Lowry (1991) note nursing's inexperience with the spiritual dimension:

> *The process of defining spiritual care and spiritual needs has been elusive at best. It is not sufficiently developed to provide students and practitioners clear direction in strategies for using it in an intervention or for measuring spirituality as a part of quality care. (p. 68)*

Clark and colleagues make clear their belief that a spiritual element is needed in nursing:

> *Spiritual well-being, the integrating aspect of human wholeness is characterized by meaning and hope. Quality care must include a spirit-to-spirit encounter between caregiver and patient. That includes the patient's acknowledgement of trust in the caregiver. (p. 68)*

From interviews, Clark and coworkers identified five major spiritual interventions as reported by patients:

1. Establishing a trusting relationship
2. Providing and facilitating a supportive environment

3. Responding sensitively to the patient's beliefs
4. Integrating spirituality into the quality assurance plan
5. Taking ownership of the nurse's key role in the health care system (pp. 74–75)

The list proves the authors' point concerning the lack of work in this arena. Many of the items are simply good nursing dictates, whether or not spirituality is involved. Indeed, spirituality may be a difficult concept to pin down because some associate it with religion, some with an attitude toward life, and others with an advanced level of human development.

Traditional Religious Influence

Not all of the renewed focus on spirituality comes from theories using a New Age paradigm. Traditional religious perspectives are also undergoing a renewed interest within the nursing community. These changes, however, are more recognized in changing nursing practices than in new theories. One such change is a new practice called parish nursing, a resurgence in nursing closely tied to a church or religious organization.

A parish nurse works for a religious group, tending to its parishioners, or in some cases to its geographic neighborhood. The parish nurse functions in much the same way that community health nurses function. About this resurgence, Smith (1991) says:

> *Parish nursing was born from the vision of Reverend Granger Westberg. Rev. Westberg worked as a hospital chaplain for many years, and his experience with nurses convinced him that they were "a national treasure." With one foot in the sciences and one foot in the humanities, Westberg believed nurses had great insight into the human condition. (p. 28)*

Smith related four generally accepted functions of the parish nurse in the new movement: (1) health educator, (2) personal health counselor, (3) trainee of volunteers, and (4) liaison with community resources (p. 28). So far, a unique *theory* of parish nursing has not been promulgated, although the functions of the role are being discussed in a practical, exploratory manner.

It appears that the religious motivation is the *context* of nursing care rather than the *content* of the role. If parish nurses were used for religious proselytizing, one would have to ask: Is religious recruitment inherent in the theory of nursing? Or is the nursing role a vehicle to put a religious worker in touch with others for the purpose of proselytizing? In a Lutheran release, Martinson (1991) quotes Westberg as saying:

. . . *a parish nurse is a much-needed "high-touch" component in the increasingly "high-tech" world of health care. In fact, insurers and government agencies should be singing the praises of parish nursing because it promotes preventive medicine, which is the least expensive form of health care. (p. 2)*

The linkage appears to be one of sympathy between the purposes of the church and nursing rather than an attempt to move the nursing ideology toward a spiritual base.

Miskelly (1995, p. 1) identifies four different models for parish nursing: (1) institutional/paid, in which the nurse is employed by a hospital of the community or a long-term facility that contracts with one or more churches; (2) institutional/volunteer, a similar position except the nurse receives no salary; (3) congregational/paid, in which the congregation directly hires the nurse; and (4) congregational/volunteer, again with the same structure but no salary involved.

Barnum (1996) notes that the parish nurse concept might be traced to a long-standing practice in this nation's many African American churches:

Another largely overlooked linkage between nursing and churches has been preserved in various African-American churches where so-called nurses, often in white uniform, take care of parishioners who may faint, suffer hysterics, or manifest other health accidents during church services. Historically, the practice probably arose in services that encouraged audience experiential phenomena. Little about the practice has been written in nursing journals, nor are these nurses always registered nurses. (pp. 12–13)

Substance Abuse Programs

One of the few arenas of care where a spiritual component is more common than not in today's health is the treatment of alcohol and drug abuse. Typically these programs are multidisciplinary, not invoking unique nursing theories. Most therapy models are based on the philosophy of Alcoholics Anonymous (AA), the first large-scale success in containing substance abuse. Bauer (1982, p. 25) claims that the AA program succeeded by taking away moral guilt, offering hope, restoring dignity, and respecting one's individuality and the need to remain in the collective society.

The keystone of the AA program was a letter by C. G. Jung to Bill W., one of the founders. In that correspondence, Jung stated that he believed abuse of alcohol to be a defective search for the spiritual. The cure for alcoholism, he said, was to be found in the spirit. Alcohol was the equivalent, on a low level, of spiritual thirst for wholeness;

it represented the search for union with God (Bauer, p. 127). Jung added:

> You see, "alcohol" in Latin is spiritus, and you use the same word for
> the highest religious experience as well as for the most depraving poison.
> The helpful formula therefore is: spiritus contra spiritum (Bauer, p. 127).

The most successful approach in treating substance abuse, the 12-step AA program and its clones in drug abuse (eg, Cocaine Anonymous and Narcotics Anonymous) grounds recovery in a relationship to a higher power. In regaining this missing sense of spirit, the abuser regains his relationship to a spiritual power. There is no attempt on the part of these programs to link to a specific church or religion, yet the notion of a higher power is taken quite literally.

Alcoholics Anonymous has taken the spiritual message to heart in an era that has pushed science as a substitute for God. Is substance abuse a natural backlash in a society seriously divorced from spiritual values? Is the rampant substance abuse of this age an ironic, thwarted search for spirit as Jung believed?

Notice the verbal imagery. Is drug *intoxication* a poor man's spiritual *intoxication*? Is it coincidence that one *gets high* on drugs just as religions point *heavenward*? Or that many drug users claim they are hooked on another reality revealed by the drug?

Whether or not one agrees that the deficit is spiritual, mere body cure (withdrawal and detoxification) seldom works. Effective rehabilitation programs discover that they must offer more than just a substance-free state. As Gold (1984, pp. 43–44) says in relation to cocaine abuse, one must fill the cocaine hours—the time that was previously filled with thinking about the drug, purchasing it, using it, hanging around with fellow abusers. AA and its imitators fill the abuse hours with a spiritual focus.

Some purists object that this substitutes one addiction for another—if one grants such a thing as addiction to religion. Others protest that the AA programs themselves constitute an alternate addiction.

Clearly the AA approach does not work for everyone. Nonbelievers, for example, may object to the spiritual orientation. Others object to the sense of personal humility demanded in the surrender to a higher power. Loners may resent the close fellowship fostered among recovering substance abusers. With all their limitations, the AA programs appear to have a higher rate of success than programs not addressing the spiritual element. The fact that the AA ideology has been widely accepted by lay and multidisciplinary professional leadership alike constitutes a strong recognition of the spiritual disease hypothesis.

Spiritualism in General Nursing Care

In addition to substance abuse programs, there is a resurgence of attention to a spiritual dimension among traditionally religious nurses. Within the Catholic tradition, Donley (1991, pp. 178–183) suggests the following spiritual responses to patients' suffering: (1) compassionate accompaniment, (2) a search for meaning in the suffering, and (3) action to remove the suffering. Here, then, is the beginning of a typology of spiritual care in relation to at least one concept: suffering. Taylor and Ferszt (1990, p. 37) discuss spiritual healing in a traditional fashion, including the value of prayer and ritualized repetitions of Biblical citations.

As with any new aspect of care, there is a need to explore the domain of spirituality before integrating it into nursing practice. The nature of spiritual care calls into question not only the nurse's knowledge but her personal qualifications to offer spiritual guidance. Nagai-Jacobson and Burkhardt (1989) and Stuart, Deckro, and Mandle (1989) raise the problem of the nurse's own spiritual deficiencies and the inadequacy of her own spiritual resources. Their objections seem only fair, for few if any schools or employers attempt to judge the nurse's spiritual qualifications, nor do many equip her for providing spiritual care.

New Age Spirituality and Nursing

We can anticipate more literature linking spiritualism and nursing as the New Age paradigm establishes itself. Dossey (1989) identifies three themes that locate the spiritual from this perspective:

1. *The metaphysics that recognizes a divine Reality substantial to the world of things and lives and minds*
2. *The psychology that finds in the soul something similar to, or even identical with, divine reality*
3. *The ethics that place the human being's final end in the knowledge of the immanent and transcendent Ground of all being—the thing is immemorial and universal (p. 27)*

Watson (1988) also considers spirituality an important component of nursing. Her ideas fluctuate between New Age and traditional:

The notion of a human soul is nothing new or original. It is, however, unusual to include it in a theory. The closest concept in psychology and nursing are concepts like self, inner self, "I," me, self-actualization, and so on. The bold attempt to acknowledge and try to incorporate a concept of the soul in a nursing theory is a reflection of an alternative position that nursing is now free to take. The new concept breaks from the traditional medical science model and is also a reflection of the scientific times. The evolution of the history and philosophy of science now allows some attention to metaphysical views that would have been unacceptable at an earlier point in time. (p.49)

Given nursing's early roots in religion, it is ironic that Watson has to search for permission to include aspects of the soul in a nursing ideology, yet it is impossible to dismiss her point. It is, indeed, the changing paradigm that encourages inclusions of spirituality. A major question not yet handled is just what nurses will *do* with the spiritual aspect of nursing where it is included and how they will be judged qualified for the work involved.

Like Watson, Quinn (1992) invokes the sense of the spiritual. Quinn has a unique conception of the nurse as a healing environment for the patient, that is, the nurse as an energetic, vibrational field, integral with the client's environment. As she says, the nurse should ask herself, "How can I become a safe space, a sacred healing vessel for this client in this moment?" (p. 27) The nurse as a healing environment facilitates the multidimensional response of a whole person in the direction of healing and interaction.

Earlier chapters have discussed methods used by Watson and Dossey. Other theorists and nurse practitioners address channeling, chakra therapy, past life regression, rebirthing, breath work, color visualization, and crystal healing. One finds much New Age phenomena in the nursing literature, and the question is one of boundary: How is the New Age nurse different from other New Age advocates? How is nursing spiritualism different from other spiritualism?

The three major New Age theories with spiritual bases or overtones are compared briefly in Table 9–1. These capsules refer to the newer materials by Watson (1988), Newman (1994), and Dossey (1995).

Prince and Reiss (1990) struggle against the constraints of the scientific world view in treating patients labeled psychotic. They note that, from a different paradigm, some of these persons might be seen as normal. In many cultures, for example, the hallucinations of shamans are taken as sacred psychological states (p. 137).

Prince and Reiss extend their perspective beyond shamanism to those labeled more frankly psychotic:

In the Western world, when psychotics speak of their subjective experiences and the supernatural beliefs which often arise from them (delusions in psychiatric parlance), they are rejected by their more rationalistic confreres. (p. 138)

The usual reaction of the psychiatrist (but not necessarily of the lay reader) to ideas such as are expressed in this piece is to dismiss them as delusional and psychotic. The psychiatrist will pay little attention to their contents, apart from noting their formal aspects and as having relevance to diagnostic criteria. . . .

Table 9-1. *Modern Spiritual Nursing Theories*

	Watson	Newman	Dossey
Content	Human soul	Mind/human consciousness	Biopsychosocio-spiritual man
Process	Caring/inter-personal	Repatterning	Doing/being
Context	Spiritual/God-ordered world	Teleological evolution of man as consciousness	Transcendent reality mediated by mind modulations of autonomic, endo-crine, immune, and neuropeptide sys-tems, but every-thing is mind
Goal	Harmony of mind-body-spirit	Evolution of consciousness	Healing/evolving to transpersonal self
Disease	Disharmony of parts	A signal of a need for change/readi-ness for higher evolution	Obstruction in evolu-tion toward next life phase
Health	Harmony	Expanding consciousness	Personal growth, expanding states of consciousness
God	The source that man strives to become like	An evolving con-sciousness of which man is a part	The ground of being to which man is similar or identical

> In dismissing these ideas as meaningless, the psychiatrist relegates
> highly significant experiences of the patient to limbo. Concerns that are
> of most importance to the patient are irrelevant to the psychiatrist. . . .
> For the psychiatrist, the explanatory model (EM) of the patient with
> respect to his or her experience is completely unrealistic and even more
> damaging, non-negotiable. (p. 141)

The new paradigm is returning us to a consideration of spiritual
matters and their place in health care. Some new models of nursing,
such as Watson's, already incorporate notions of spirituality; others
are certain to follow. New Age practices are seeping into everyday

nursing practice. A nurse and social worker recently recounted to me an experience in which nurses and patients were encouraged to attend brief sessions of meditation and stress relaxation in the New Age venue. One patient, who had apparently never considered that nurses experience stresses and vulnerability, found it virtually an epiphany.

Most of the nursing theories that look at spiritualism from a New Age paradigm come from a holistic perception. Indeed, for those that adopt a transpersonal psychology as a base, spiritual development may be a natural phase of self-evolution beyond the more traditional stopping point at self-actualization.

ETHICS IN NURSING

When one turns from spirituality to ethics (at least as the notion appears in nursing), there is a radical shift in orientation. We move away from the idea of lifting the human spirit upward to an ideology, often with a sense of burden, always with a sense of duty. The study of ethics has always had importance to nursing theory because the majority of nursing theories prescribe how the nurse ought to act. (We are into rule setting here, obligations, dictates—not joyful uplifting of spirit.)

Most theorists, in their own way, identify the assumptions out of which the *good* nurse ought to act. Even theorists who write descriptive theory, such as Benner (1984), express values. Much of her data consists of *excellent* exemplars, that is, practice anecdotes already judged to be good.

Sometimes the link between a theory and its underlying ethical system is not as tight as the author might wish. Although New Age holistic theories instill the spiritual as an intrinsic aspect, the older theories had more difficulty integrating ethics into their theory components. It is not unusual for a reader to find a theorist proclaiming an ethical underpinning only to discover that the espoused ethical stance is superimposed rather than intrinsic to the theory. Some would argue this to be the case for Roy's (1989) stimulus–response theory. The espoused value system seems to be a slogan rather than a principle that drives the theory. Indeed, Roy can hardly be faulted for the failure because her stimulus–response theory represents the most removed view from man as spirit.

Ethical Quandaries

Unlike the spiritual nursing focus, the ethical focus fixates on problems. Often they involve exigencies of the practice setting. Issues often arise from tensions between cost control and quality of care or between quality of life and technology. Ethical positions look at the nurse from a behavioral viewpoint, namely, considering what she ought to *do*. Ethics has a function of rule giving, behavior controlling. From this perspective the practice arena engenders an ever-increasing number of ethical questions and few definitive answers.

The rule-giving orientation produces ethical quandaries when changes in the environment confront people with new situations lacking ethical precedents. The linkage with law rears its head, as decisions about new procedures and practices slowly are codified into laws and regulations. Today's health care environment is rampant with examples of such equivocal situations. This week's paper ponders the ethics of a 63-year-old woman who just became a mother, giving birth to a child from a donor egg fertilized with her husband's sperm. The issue was not concerning the ethics of donor eggs (that was last year's ethical quandary). This time, the dilemma was the woman's age and whether it was right for a woman to give birth to a child when she might not live out its full childhood/adolescence.

Sometimes the issue is economics. New technologies and new health care products have increased the range of health care options, yet the cost of these innovations often exceeds the ability of society to pay for them. Society must decide which options will be developed and which will not—a decision governing bodies are reluctant to make.

One of the major problems from the ethical viewpoint is how to resolve the tension between a continuously developing science whose technology prolongs life versus the cost to society. This conflict occurs only when one accepts two normative sets of values: (1) the medical ideology that prolonged life of any quality is a prime value, and (2) the social-economic preference not to place additional fiscal investment in the health care of people.

A nurse holding a New Age ideology might find this problem beside the point. She might argue that prolonging life is not itself a very important goal, that, indeed, it might obstruct the soul development of persons who have elected to experience lives cut short. She might consider the markers of life and death to be rather inconsequential in the longer view of a soul's development over various lifetimes.

The point to be made here is that ethics are very much tied to a society's and nurse's world view. One's accepted world paradigm will dictate what nursing theories will appeal and which will not. In the past era, when most nurses in this culture shared the same world, even different ethical positions could be discussed from a common beginning point. That is no longer the case.

Quality of Life and Death Decisions

Even under the older scientific ideology (that is still predominant), changes are coming about in ethical values. The increased respect for quality of life is a good example. Quality of life is the first value to confront head-on the medical assumption the preservation of life is always to be desired. On the whole, nurses are more comfortable than physicians with decisions to allow certain patients to die. Now patients and their families, in increasing numbers, are demanding their rights in that decision-making process. What was once settled by an authoritarian physician has become a negotiation in which many persons have a stake and in which "life at any cost" is no longer seen as the right answer.

The ethical dilemma is complicated by the legal issue, that is, the vulnerability of those who take measures to stop or prevent life-preserving therapy. The court position is slow to change, following, not leading normative practices in the society. Assisted suicide is a major issue at present, with the Dutch example held up as humanitarian by those who defend this position.

Equity in Health Care

The issue of equity is also problematic in the ethical decision-making paradigm. Most reasonable people would agree that health care should be equitable, yet what constitutes equity is not so simple. One party's equity is another's deprivation. What represents equity when parents from different social strata, with different means, compete for a scarce resource, say a liver for a dying child? What about the rights of a financially stressed surrogate mother versus the rights of the wealthy contracting father? What about the rights of their child? How is equity acted out when a patient with a terminal condition seeks to discontinue life support in the face of family opposition? What is equitable about a reduced population of young people carrying the Social Security tax burden for a disproportionate number of old and old-old in the general population? This does not even touch on issues of equity for those who are denied health care access because they lack the ability to pay. The problems of equity expand to tomes with very little effort.

The cases and causes are numerous, but in each example one asks: Who decides? Who pays? Who has rights? Who has obligations? What is justice? The problem in making most of these decisions is that the choice does not involve choosing between right and wrong, good and bad; instead it involves choosing between opposing goods. When one discusses morality in terms of rights, justice, and equity, the argument hinges on the older world view.

When Nurses Confront Ethical Issues

Ethical issues arise for the nurse in the old perspective in several ways. Zablow's (1984) study reported nurses being caught between physician demands and actions they believed to be right for the patient. In such situations, the nurses felt pressured to yield to the physician's decree because of his perceived power in the institution.

Additionally, some nurses feared that their organizations would not support them for ethical stands taken on disputable issues. Unfortunately, some of these nurses may have been right. In these circumstances, the nurses felt powerless to exercise control, even over their own behavior.

In regular nursing practice, issues having ethical implications surface with regularity. They include but are not limited to: do not resuscitate practices; management for suspected child, wife, and elder abuse; patient's right to informed consent; patient's right to privacy and confidentiality; and the patient's right to die. These examples are only some of the more blatant issues.

Nor is it possible for the nurse using a holistic, New Age theory to avoid dealing with these issues because she is in a world of action just as much as is the nurse holding an older ideology. Of course, none of these issues can be altogether resolved by a policy statement. Reasonable people may disagree on principles and even on actions where they agree on principles.

Sometimes the real moral dilemmas arising for nurses relate not so much to hard ethical choices but to options forgone because of limitations on staff and resources. Financial stringency may be necessary for an institution's survival, but many nurses face quandaries of conscience when they see needy patients turned away because of inability to pay. Others face moral dilemmas when the situation simply allows them insufficient time to meet critical patient needs.

Institutional Solutions

Most institutions attempt to deal with ethical problems by the committee route. An ethics committee decides on the best action in serious, ambiguous cases with ethical and legal overtones. Such committees function to prevent arbitrary and premature decision-making in complex cases. Even with a committee, however, there may be honest moral disagreements on the best way to handle a given problem. The use of deliberative, committee decision-making offers some legal protection. Legal judgments may be requested in particularly complex circumstances.

An institutional review board serves as another clearing house for ethical problems—those that arise in medical, nursing, and other research endeavors using patients as subjects. Even though such committees are comprised of people holding different beliefs, joint deliberation has merit. The quality of decision-making certainly is improved by a thoughtful, contemplative process.

The interplay of ethics and research has always been an important issue for nurses. Munhall (1988), for example, discusses the way in which the therapeutic imperative (patient advocacy) must take precedence over the research imperative. In Munhall's view, informed consent must be seen as dynamic and ongoing, hence invalidated if the circumstances under which the consent was obtained change.

Ethical Guides

Every nurse should understand the norms of her society regarding ethical judgments. This is true whether or not the nurse personally comes from the same ideology. Probably the greatest change in recent years has been the growing involvement of people in their own health care decisions. Acceptance of the patient's right to participate in full and informed decision-making regarding his condition, prognosis, and treatment is a relatively new value. The President's Commission for the Study of Ethical Problems in Medicine and Biomedical and Behavioral Research (1982, pp. 15–68) stressed patient autonomy as one of its hallmarks. This reflects a clear change in the normative society's way of perceiving the relationship between patient and health care professional.

The Judicial Council of the American Medical Association (1984) wrestled with the ethics of medical practice, addressing numerous issues of complexity ranging from ethical business practices for physicians to physician–patient relations. Ethical business practices are at issue as more physicians are becoming partial owners in care delivery systems. Physician–patient relations have always been problematic, and, in this respect, the Judicial Council formulated criteria for patient access to scarce resources in cases of necessary rationing. The document (1984) stated:

> Limited health care resources should be allocated efficiently and on the basis of fair, acceptable and humanitarian criteria. Priority should be given to persons who are most likely to be treated successfully or have long term benefit. Social worth is not an appropriate criterion. (p. 3)

The nursing profession lacks such a judicial board, but it has a published code of ethics. The American Nurses Association's (1985) *Code for Nurses* provides guidelines concerning nurses' obligations to patients, colleagues, and the larger society. It does not, except in the broadest of terms, address specific ethical dilemmas such as access to health for the uninsured and homeless, abortion, do not resuscitate orders, medical experimentation, distribution of scarce health resources, or allocation of expensive technology. Nor can it tell the nurse what to do in particular situations. The code is a useful guide, but ethical decisions still need to be puzzled out in light of the unique situational variables in each case. The code falls prey to the flaws of attempting to dictate concrete, specific actions by generalized rules of behavior.

A PHILOSOPHICAL OVERVIEW OF ETHICS

In addition to the practical differences in the two notions of valuing most dominant in nursing (the traditional ethics focus and emerging notions of spirituality), one can consider the differences among ethical positions as from a philosophic approach. Figure 9–1 presents some of the possible ethical positions.

The first differentiation is between a philosophy of *determinism* and one espousing human *freedom*. In determinism, all things happen in terms of antecedents. If one knew what had happened in the past, one could predict a present action. In this belief system, man has no free will; consequently, there is no such things as ethics. If all choices are the inevitable result of earlier events, then one cannot be morally accountable for his acts. To allow for ethics, there must first be some freedom of choice; one must be able to choose right over wrong.

Among theories that espouse human freedom of choice and will, there are two positions. In one formulation, *ethical choice* exists; in the other, *moral skepticism* holds forth. The latter position claims that, although people are free to choose, the choices they make are not influenced by ethics. Moral choice is illusory in moral skepticism; ethics is an empty word. People choose for their own benefit but not on the basis of what is good or bad.

Among positions that support the existence of ethics in choice-making, we can make yet another differentiation, one based on the way in which something is known to be ethical. Here one asks, what makes an act ethical? Again there are two possible answers, *teleological* or *deontological*.

Teleology refers to the end, result, or goal. Teleological systems place ethics in one of two final loci (making another set of options). Some teleological positions judge an act ethical according to its *intentions*. Others judge an act ethical according to its *consequences*. The same act might be ethical in one system and unethical in another. Suppose a professor passed a borderline student to be kind (inten-

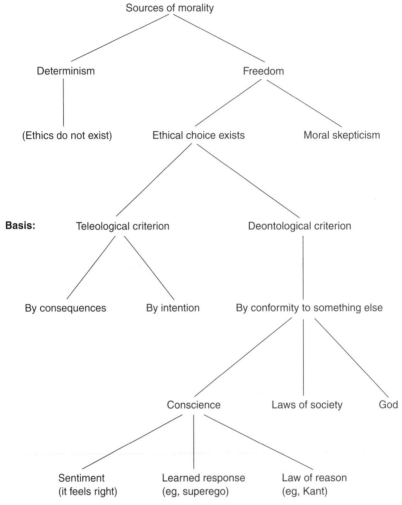

Figure 9–1. *Why good people disagree on ethical issues.*

tion). Suppose further, that the student's ignorance in the subject matter caused the death of a patient (consequence). The act of the professor (passing her) would be judged differently by persons holding these alternate teleological positions.

The deontological position judges an act neither by its intentions nor its consequences. Instead, it judges an act to be ethical based on its conformity with something else. The something else, as you might suspect, varies from philosophy to philosophy. Three common options might be (1) the *laws* of the society, (2) *God* (or His revealed word, however conceptualized), or (3) one's *conscience*.

Conscience illustrates the complexity. The problem is that different consciences dictate different acts. Further, there are many different interpretations of conscience. Some see it is a *learned response*. One might, for example, place Freud's internalization of the superego in this category. A second interpretation of conscience might be that it is the *law of reason*. Here one might refer to logical rules like Kant's categorical imperative (1986, pp. 53–125). Another interpretation finds conscience in *sentiment*; the inner voice theory might represent this view—whatever feels right.

For one last differentiation, let us look at the notion of sentiment. If one responds to an inner voice, it is still possible to ask how that inner voice makes its decisions. Does it intuit that certain *rules* are good, for example, never tell a lie, do not commit murder? Or does the sentiment function to judge each act separately? In the latter case, it might be right to murder in one case (when the axe murderer is attacking one's children) but not in another case.

For a different philosophical perspective on ethics, look at Bandman and Bandman (1995) who discuss the following theories of modern morality: egoism, rational paternalism, altruism, the social contract, utilitarianism, universal moral principles, voluntarism, duty-based ethics, Marxism, existentialism, relativism and subjectivism, hedonism, stoicism, and other categories.

This rather incomplete analysis of the nature of ethics and the meaning ethics holds for persons of different philosophies is intended only to make the nurse cognizant of the complexity of the subject. People of good will, all of whom identify themselves as moral, may disagree in good faith.

COMPARING PERSPECTIVES

The inherent conflict between a rule-oriented, rights-and-duties concept of ethics and a larger spiritual perspective might shed light on the ongoing dispute in nursing between the perspectives of Kohlberg and Gilligan on moral development. Kohlberg's (1981) classificatory system for *moral development* evolved under the more traditional conception of ethics. The system typifies the view of ethics described here: rule-bound, dealing with concepts of justice and equity. Numerous nurse researchers used his schema, but women in general and nurses in particular did not test well under Kohlberg's highly formal and abstract system.

The premise for Kohlberg's system was challenged by Gilligan (1982), claiming that female morality is derived from personal relationships rather than abstract concepts. Although Gilligan certainly does not come from a New Age ideology, her work shows that the notion of ethics need not be limited to the older models.

SUMMARY

Ethics and the new spiritualism often arise from different conceptions of the world. They present different problems, goals, values, and approaches. What they share is a focus on values and the need to negotiate between personal beliefs and societal norms. Nursing has had an interesting historical love affair with spirituality. Nursing had its origin in religion. Much of our early history concerns nurses dedicated to the profession because of a religious commitment— usually to a codified belief system set in the context of a given religion.

Along the way, the religious origins of nursing were lost, some would say systematically sacrificed in the name of professionalism and the scientific method. Even nursing schools sponsored by religious institutions frequently failed to include aspects of spirituality in the curriculum of care giving in the 1940s and 1950s. In the practice setting, spirituality became the domain of the chaplain not the nurse.

In modern times, morality again reared its head, spurred by the ethical quandaries and legal problems created by the advancement of technology and the impositions of a lawsuit-prone society. The study of ethics returned to nursing as an administrative/legal necessity. The focus was on helping patients make difficult care decisions or protecting the nurse, physician, and the institution from malfeasance.

Newer theories of nursing, those cast in a New Age ideology, present a view of morality based in spiritual/developmental values. At present, both of these aspects (ethics and spirituality) are at play in nursing. Although they are not necessarily at odds with each other, they represent different perspectives on the underlying moral concerns.

REFERENCES

American Medical Association. (1984). *Current opinions of the Judicial Council of the American Medical Association.* Chicago: Author.
American Nurses Association. (1985). *Code for nurses with interpretive statement.* Washington, DC: Author.
Bandman, E. L., & Bandman, B. (1995). *Nursing ethics through the life span* (3rd ed.). Norwalk, CT: Appleton & Lange.
Barnum, B. S. (1996). *Spirituality in nursing: From traditional to New Age.* New York: Springer.

Bauer, J. (1982). *Alcoholism and women.* Toronto: Inner City Books.

Benner, P. (1984). *From novice to expert: Excellence and power in clinical nursing practice.* Menlo Park, CA: Addison-Wesley.

Clark, C., Cross, J. R., Deane, D. M., & Lowry, L. W. (1991, April). Spirituality: Integral to quality care. *Holistic Nursing Process, 3,* 67–76.

Donley, R. (1991, April). Spiritual dimensions of health care: Nursing's mission. *Nursing & Health Care, 4,* 178–183.

Dossey, B. M. (1989). The transpersonal self and states of consciousness. In B. M. Dossey, L. Keegan, L. G. Kolkmeier, & C. E. Guzzetta (Eds.), *Holistic health promotion: A guide for practice* (pp. 23–50). Rockville, MD: Aspen.

Dossey, B. M., Keegan, L. G., Guzzetta, C. E., & Kolkmeier, L. G., (1995). *Holistic nursing: A handbook for practice* (2nd ed.). Gaithersburg, MD: Aspen.

Gilligan, C. (1982). *In a different voice: Psychological theory and women's development.* Cambridge, MA: Harvard University Press.

Gold, M. S. (1984). *800-Cocaine.* New York, Bantam Books.

Hover-Kramer, D. (1989, May). Creating a context for self-healing: The transpersonal perspective. *Holistic Nursing Practice, 3,* 27–34.

Kant, I. (1986). Foundations of the metaphysics of morals. In E. Behler (Ed.), *Immanuel Kant: Philosophical writings* (pp. 52–125). New York: Continuum.

Kohlberg, L. (1981). *The meaning and measurement of moral development.* Worcester, MA: Clark University Press.

Longway, I. (1970, February/March). Toward a philosophy of nursing. *Journal of Adventist Education, 3,* 20–27.

Martinson, V. (1991, October). *Founder of parish nurse movement urges return to "high-touch" health care for a "high-tech" world.* [News Release]. Park Ridge, IL: Lutheran General Health Care System, pp. 1–4.

Miskelly, S. (1995). A parish nursing model: Applying the community health nursing process in a church community. *Journal of Community Health Nursing, 1,* 1–14.

Munhall, P. L. (1988). Ethical considerations in qualitative research. *Western Journal of Nursing Research, 2,* 150–162.

Nagai-Jacobson, M. G., & Burkhardt, M. A. (1989, May). Spirituality: Cornerstone of holistic nursing practice. *Holistic Nursing Practice, 3,* 18–26.

Newman, M. A. (1989). The spirit of nursing. *Holistic Nursing Practice, 3,* 1–6.

Newman, M. A. (1994). *Health as expanding consciousness.* New York: National League for Nursing Press.

President's Commission for the Study of Ethical Problems in Medicine and Biomedical and Behavioral Research. (1982, October). *Making health care decisions, Vol. 1: Report.* Washington, DC: U.S. Government Printing Office.

Prince, R. H., & Reiss, M. (1991, September). Psychiatry and the irrational: Does our scientific world view interfere with the adaptation of psychotics? *Psychiatric Journal of the University of Ottawa, 3,* 137–143.

Quinn, J. F. (1992, July). Holding sacred space: The nurse as healing environment. *Holistic Nursing Practice, 4,* 26–36.

Roy, C. (1989). The Roy adaptation model. In J. Riehl-Sisca, *Conceptual models for nursing practice* (3rd ed., pp. 105–114). New York: Appleton-Century-Crofts.

Smith, P. K. (1991, Summer). The parish nurse. *The Communique, Quarterly Publication of the Wisconsin League for Nursing, Inc, 2,* 28–29.

Stuart, E. M., Deckro, J. D., & Mandle, C. L. (1989, May). Spirituality in health and healing: A clinical program. *Holistic Nursing Practice, 3,* 35–46.

Taylor, P. B., & Ferszt, G. G. (1990, July). Spiritual healing. *Holistic Nursing Practice, 4,* 32–38.

Watson, J. (1988). *Nursing: Human science and human care: A theory of nursing.* New York: National League for Nursing.

Zablow, R. J. (1984). *Preparing students for the moral dimension of professional nursing practice: A protocol for nurse educators.* Unpublished dissertation, Teachers College, Columbia University, New York.

10 *Principle, Interpretation, and Method*

USE OF ANALYTICAL DEVICES IN UNDERSTANDING THEORY

Chapters 1 and 2 presented certain analytical devices for theory analysis: (1) using commonplaces to define theory elements, (2) determining the level of theory development (descriptive or explanatory), (3) determining the boundaries that discriminate nursing from nonnursing acts, (4) locating the theory on a patient–interaction–nurse continuum, (5) recognizing relevant underlying assumptions, and (6) recognizing slogans and selective perception. Three additional analytical devices are presented in this chapter: description of theory as to (1) principle, (2) interpretation, and (3) method. This system may be used instead of analysis by content, process, context, and goals if the reader finds it useful. If it seems too complex, the other method is satisfactory for making most significant differentiations.

PRINCIPLE

Every nursing theory is based on one or more dominant principles. A *principle* is the crux of a theory, an idea that is essential for stating or explaining it. Depending on the author's way of thinking, a principle may be presented as a starting point or as an ending point. Hall (1966) and Orlando (1990) illustrate these different approaches. Hall arrives at her basic principle of self-mastery at the end of a chain of reasoning, and she places it at the end of her article. Orlando, in contrast, asserts her principle by the second page, stating:

> *It is, therefore, exceedingly important for the nurse to distinguish be-*
> *tween her understanding of general principles and the meanings which*
> *she must discover in the immediate nursing situation in order to help*
> *the patient. In making the distinction, the nurse first attempts to under-*
> *stand the meaning to the patient in a time and place context of what*
> *she observes and how she can exercise her professional function in*
> *relation to it. (p. 2)*

Orlando used the rest of her book to clarify and explain the principle, through more complete description and numerous examples of how it functions. Most authors follow one of these two patterns: (1) working toward a final discovery of the principle(s), or (2) stating the principle(s) and then explaining the ramifications.

Because nursing theories usually deal with both patients and nursing acts, it is not unusual to find *complementary principles*, one residing in the patient and one in the nursing act. For example, Hall's principle of self-mastery in the patient is complementary to the principle of mirroring in the nursing act. Similarly, Orlando's nurse interprets to the patient what she thinks his behavior means, and the patient confirms or disconfirms its meaning.

Not all principles rest in the patient or the nursing act. Some principles rest in other aspects of the situation. For example, King's (1981) principles (action, transaction, and interaction) are found in the interaction rather than in either the patient or nurse.

A theory may have one or several main principles. One should identify each key principle of a theory, then consider the *nature* of each principle. Compare, for example, Hall's patient-based principle of *self-mastery* with Levine's (1971) patient-based principle of *adaptation*. For Hall, the principle rests in the agent himself. (Hall said that the patient *chooses* ill behavior or well behavior.) This sort of principle is termed *actional*: the principle is part of the agent. Self-mastery (for Hall) can occur in a patient with very little control over his own body or environment. Indeed, self-mastery may take place (or fail to take place) in favorable or unfavorable circumstances. Actional principles are found in human drives, motives, needs, or intentions.

Levine's adaptation principle, on the other hand, is located in the interaction of agent and circumstance. Adaptation means a constant adjustment of the individual to his changing environment (circumstances). This sort of principle is termed *reflexive*. Reflexive principles in nursing often are characterized by states of homeostasis, equilibrium, or exchange.

The difference between actional and reflexive principles can be illustrated by contrasting two additional theories. Flaskerud, Halloran, Janken, Lund, and Zetterlund (1979) present a nursing theory that is unusual in that it is based on observation of *what is* instead of *what ought to be*. In multiple observations of nurses working in diverse settings, the authors found two consistent principles at work: *avoidance* and *distancing*. These are actional principles because they describe behaviors located in the agent (in this case, the nurse). The behaviors were exhibited consistently without being altered in kind by the settings or patients involved. The actions were *by* the nurse, *for* the nurse.

In contrast to Flaskerud and colleagues, Orlando has a reflexive principle. The nurse observes a specific patient behavior that she believes has significance. She identifies the behavior and verbally reflects it back to the patient with her interpretation of what the behavior means. The patient then corrects any misinterpretations before the nurse acts on them. The nurse cannot make a final judgment without the patient's input. When the behavior is called to the patient's attention, if he had not previously recognized the behavior, this mirroring back enables him to reflect on the behavior and its meaning. Interaction theories such as Orlando's often involve reflexive principles.

There are two other types of principle: *comprehensive* and *simple*. The comprehensive principle explains a phenomenon by reference to a larger whole. For example, one might explain why a child is unable to perform a given psychomotor task by reference to the principle of *learning readiness*. Learning readiness is a larger notion than the specific task failure that it explains. The same principle of learning readiness might explain hundreds of other task failures as well as task achievements. The principle of learning readiness is overarching, larger, and more comprehensive than those specific instantiations of it.

One might, on the other hand, have explained the child's failure in the psychomotor task by reference to the absence of the requisite series of stimulus–response patterns in his behavior. Here the explanation directs attention to component parts of the phenomenon rather than to some overarching whole. Principles of this sort are termed simple. A simple principle explains a phenomenon by reference to its component parts (ie, to its elemental building bricks). To explain a human being as so many interacting atoms uses a simple principle, whereas to explain man as an instantiation of a moving life process uses a comprehensive principle.

Rogers (1970) uses comprehensive principles. In her early work, she explains the human being by reference to the principle of reciprocy, a principle that relates man to his environmental field (p. 97), that is, a larger entity encompassing the human and the environment. Like Rogers's theory, Newman's (1994) has a comprehensive principle, identifying health, the goal of nursing, as the expansion of consciousness (p. xxiii). But expansion of consciousness does not simply mean learning new things or becoming more adept at one's cognitive or affective functions. Instead, it involves actual change in what one is, in the patterning that is the essence of a one's being. The goal of nursing is to move a person toward becoming, toward a higher level of existence and awareness. The principle of expansion of consciousness represents a greater whole than the present person.

Roy's (1989) theory, in contrast to those of Rogers and Newman, uses a simple principle, explaining man on the basis of stimulus, response, and adaptation levels. The stimulus and response are parts of the phenomenon being explained; they do not constitute a whole larger than the human being.

In summary, principles may be given as starting or ending points of a theory; they may reside in the patient, nurse, or situation; and they may be actional, reflexive, comprehensive, or simple, a system of analysis borrowed from McKeon (n.d.; 1954). A principle is a fundamental or basic concept with an explanatory function, revealing the basis on which the theory is built. It is the fulcrum on which the rest of the theory depends.

INTERPRETATION

To determine interpretation in McKeon's system, one asks: What is reality (or the reality of the phenomenon under consideration) for the author? This is identical to what we have earlier called context. Examining the meanings given to the major terms of the theory provides the best clue. The essence of a theory's subject matter falls either within human experience (phenomenal) or beyond human experience (transcendental).

Where the theory places the subject of nursing within human experience (phenomenal), it is possible to label it as either *existential* or *essential*. In an existential theory, the subject matter of nursing rests in the human agent's acts, ideas, or impulses. A nursing theory based on empathy or personal power, for example, would be interpreted as existential. Both empathy and power can be experienced directly, and both can be perceived as primarily personal to and for the agent experiencing them.

Paterson and Zderad's (1988) world is existential:

> When I, nurse, respond in the arena of my lived nursing world, I respond to a particular person in this "here and now" with all my background and all my anticipation of the future. (p. 57)

> *To me, a nurse is a being, becoming through intersubjectively calling and responding in her suffering, joyous, struggling, chaotic humanness, always trying beyond the possible while never completely free from ignoble personal wants. (p. 56)*

In contrast, an essential interpretation is one in which the nursing phenomenon is explained by reference to the circumstance in which it occurs. For example, Arakelian (1980) has an essential interpretation when she proposes nursing actions based on a patient's locus of control. The patient with an internal locus of control sees himself in control of his own fate (or the events in his life); the patient with an external locus of control sees things as happening to him—by luck, fate, or through acts of a powerful other. Arakelian recommends shifting the patient with an external locus of control toward a perception of internal control so as to make him assume responsibility for his health and therapy. This theory has an essential interpretation because what constitutes the underlying reality is the patient's relationship to the world (controlling the world or being controlled by it).

It may be difficult to decide whether a phenomenal theory is existential or essential. Because nursing inevitably occurs in an extant setting, the reader may have a tendency to view all theories as essential. In assigning an interpretive category, one must look for predominance of perspective rather than for an absolute. One asks, how does this theorist really see the world of nursing? What perspective dominates? What meaning underlies the theorist's selected terms? Many nurse theorists use the same terms, so it is important to examine the meaning of terms within a given theory. Subtle shifts of meaning for the same term take place from one theorist to another.

Hall, for example, might appear, at first glance, to have an essentialist theory. There is interaction with circumstance on the part of the nurse; she interacts with the patient and his body. But the theory is existential, not essential. The *significant* world is the world of person (ie, the world of mind, awareness, and mastery). Levine's concept of nursing, on the other hand, is context imbedded; the patient's adaptations involve response to and interaction with the environment. The same is true of the nurse; her environment is the patient himself, and the nature of her conservation measures depends on an accurate reading of his responses. Levine's theory is essential in its interpretation.

Because nursing is an applied discipline, it might be expected that all theories would use one of the phenomenal approaches to interpretation, but that is not the case. Transcendental interpretations (beyond experience) consist of two types: *ontic* and *entitative*. The ontic interpretation sees the nursing reality as larger than life, and hence, *above* direct experience; the entitative interpretation sees real-

ity as *reductive* (ie, consisting of units that are microscopic or micro-
cosmic). To describe human behavior by reference to nerve cells and
synapses is an *entitative* interpretation. To describe human behavior
by reference to life phases, or an evolving consciousness, on the
other hand, is *ontic*. Neither the nerve cell nor the life phase can be
experienced in itself.

Neuman (1980, p. 120) exemplifies an entitative approach to
nursing theory by describing the human in his multicomponents: (1)
basic structure and energy resources (eg, genetic structure, response
pattern, organ strength, ego strength), (2) individual intervening variables (eg, basic structure idiosyncrasies, natural and learned resistance, time or encounter with stressor), (3) stressors (similarly broken
into component types), (4) lines of resistance, and (5) various other
perceived elements. Neuman's theory is entitative because it describes man (and nursing) by reference to simple elements.

Jones (1978) also has a transcendental, entitative theory. She
describes reality as follows:

> *Syntoxic responses trigger messengers that act as tissue tranquilizers,*
> *creating a passive tolerance that permits a kind of peaceful coexistence*
> *with aggressors. Catatoxic messengers stimulate active efforts to destroy*
> *the aggressor. Among the best-known syntoxic messengers are the anti-*
> *inflammatory corticoids. . . . (p. 1902)*

Syntoxic and catatoxic response-triggering messengers are
smaller than that which they explain and are not directly accessible
to human experience.

One may contrast this with the ontic interpretation of Newman (1994):

> *The last stage is absolute consciousness, which has been equated with*
> *love. In this state all opposites are reconciled. This kind of love embraces*
> *all experience equally and unconditionally; pain as well as pleasure,*
> *failure as well as success, ugliness as well as beauty, disease as well as*
> *non-disease. (p. 48)*

Here the human being is described, not by reference to a reality
of diverse components, but by finding the *whole* of being, in this
case, participation in full consciousness. Newman's interpretation
is ontic because what is *most real* for her is this transcendental state
of being, most real even though most of us have yet to experience it.

Watson (1988), like Newman, embodies an ontic interpretation
of man and reality:

> *My conception of life and personhood is tied to notions that one's soul*
> *possesses a body that is not confined by objective space and time. The*
> *lived world of the experiencing person is not distinguished by external*

and internal notions of time and space, but shapes its own time and space, which is unconstrained by linearity. Notions of personhood, then transcend the here and now, and one has the capacity to coexist with past, present, future, all at once. (p. 45)

A nursing theory is valid to the extent that it represents what is most truly real to the theorist. If the reader, however, does not perceive Watson's transcendental world as the most real characteristic of life, or even of nursing, then she is not likely to accept the theory. Similarly, Roy's theory will not be accepted if the nurse cannot buy stimulus–response patterns as most representative of the nursing world.

In a nursing theory, the interpretation reveals the setting so to speak, the screen (or world) on which (or within which) the theory is played out. Interpretations may be ontic, entitative, essential, or existential, and they reflect an author's underlying perception of the character of nursing. They point out the location of the *real world of nursing* for each theorist. There can be differences between a person's view of the larger reality and the view of the nursing world. For example, one may believe in a transcendental self as portrayed in many New Age theories, yet think that this is not the appropriate subject matter (ie, world) for the acts of nursing.

METHOD

Not only can a theorist be characterized by her principles and interpretation, but she can be classified by the way in which she reasons. In examining how various theorists move from their givens (principles) to their conclusions, different thought patterns emerge. These can be termed *dialectic, logistic, problematic,* and *operational.* McKeon (n.d.) describes these patterns in the following way:

Among the numerous semantic schemes that have been used in philosophy, one persistent and useful organization has been built about differences of method. For all their ambiguity the differences between dialogue or the dialectical method, debate or the operational method, proof or the logistic method, and inquiry or the problematic method were stated in ancient philosophy, have run through histories of restatement and modification, and are still operative in contemporary philosophy (p. 3).

In analyzing method in a given theory presentation, one looks for the dominant thought pattern. For most well-developed theory statements, it is possible to identify a dominant thought pattern even if patterns are somewhat mixed.

Dialectic Method

The *dialectic* method works by taking as its perspective a whole that organizes everything else. The whole, however described, governs the relationships and provides coherence to the parts. The overarching organization is emphasized in this mode of thought. All components are parts of a larger whole, a whole that is different from and greater than a mere summation of those parts. The parts, taken together, do not exhaust the whole; the whole organizes the parts.

Reasoning in the dialectic method moves by *assimilation*. Contradictory views are resolved by progression to a higher level from which the contradictions are seen as compatible components in a larger unity. This form of reasoning assimilates apparently contradictory assertions into a higher statement—higher in that it encompasses the truth embodied in each of the lower statements (Fig. 10–1).

In nursing theory, Rogers (1990) and Newman (1994) are dialectic thinkers. Nursing is explained by reference to broader principles, those that explain the human being. People, in turn, are explained by principles that characterize the universe. For Newman, that universe, all of being, is an overarching expanding consciousness in which humans participate.

Rogers's (1990) reality is revealed in her dialectic principles (ever-expanding explanatory concepts). Her principle of integrality, for example, is the assimilation of human and environmental fields; her principle of helicy assimilates integrality with continuous innovative, unpredictable, increasing diversity (p. 8). The welding of

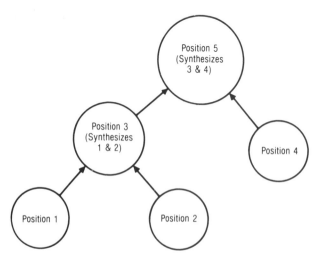

Figure 10–1. *Pattern in dialectic method.*

seemingly contrary fields is easy to identify in Roger's (1970) older book:

> If the process of life is to be studied and understood, normal and pathological processes must be treated on a basis of complete equality. . . . The life process possesses its own unity. It is inseparable from the environment. The characteristics of the life process are those of the whole. (p. 85)

Many nurses from an Anglo-American culture are not familiar with a dialectic mode of thought; hence a philosophy of this sort sounds strange at first reading. Rogers has both an unusual interpretation (eg, energy fields and resonant wave patterns), and a less-used methodology (dialectic).

Smith (1981, pp. 43–50) applies a dialectic method to more common subject matter in examining the goal of nursing: health. She identifies four different conceptualizations of health: the clinical model, the role-performance model, the adaptive model, and the eudaimonistic model. Each model is subsumed within the next, more comprehensive model. Achievement of clinical health (physiologic, biologic health) is subsumed in the role-performance model that incorporates other elements in its goal of achieving social functioning. In turn, the role-performance model is subsumed in the adaptive model, which incorporates social function into a larger notion of growth and development in interaction with one's environment. Similarly, the adaptive model is subsumed in the eudaimonistic model, whose goal incorporates growth and development within a larger goal of self-actualization.

Logistic Method

The *logistic* mode of thought moves in an opposite direction from the dialectic. In this case, the whole is not used to organize the parts, but the parts are used to explain and organize the whole. A system, event, or entity is described by reference to its parts and their interrelationships.

Reasoning in the logistic mode moves by *construction*, as piece is added to piece and relationship added to relationship. Logistic thinkers often are called system builders because their method creates a structure that resembles a geometric proof, with more and more complex rules or relations being produced in the system. Each complex rule (or component) can be broken down into the less complex rules (or components) from which it was derived. These rules in turn can be broken into simpler and simpler, and finally self-evident, rules. The mode of thought moves from the complex phenomenon to be explained to the simpler component parts of which it is comprised (Fig. 10–2).

In chemistry, all physical objects are characterized by reduction to basic elements and their interrelationships. Attention is placed on how parts interrelate with each other, how this atom of hydrogen relates to that atom of oxygen. Unlike the dialectic mode, the logistic method does not focus on how a given part fits in relation to the whole; logistic method is not concerned with assertions about how this particular atom fits into the universe.

The logistic mode is evidenced in a search for relationships—spatial, temporal, and causal. Even if the content of a logistic system becomes extensive (eg, nuclear physics explaining the whole physical universe), the construct still rests on an analysis of the parts and their relationships, not on an analysis from the viewpoint of the whole. A computer is the perfect example of a logistic system because the interface of elements is clearly established. One cannot strike the wrong key and get the function wanted. Relationships are defined and programmed and comprise the whole.

The logistic method of thought is popular in the Anglo-American culture, and many writers of nursing theory use it. Hardy (1973) typifies the logistic approach to theory development:

> *Laws are well-grounded and empirically confirmed hypotheses. They state a constant relation among two or more variables, each representing (at least partly and indirectly) a property of concrete systems. An example of a law is $E = Mc^2$. In the psycho-social area few, if any, laws exist. Laws are propositions asserting universal connection between properties. Hypotheses are much less well established (ie, have less empirical support) than laws.*
>
> *Statements on the highest level of generality are laws and axioms. Statements on a lower level of generality (theorems, hypotheses) can be*

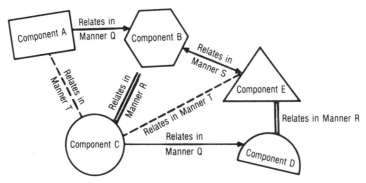

Figure 10–2. *Pattern in logistic method.*

deduced from laws. The reason for deducing these statements is to permit the general statements to be tested. In such a deductive system, high level statements can be falsified by the falsification of lower level (deduced) statements. (p. 15)

The adoption of mathematical terms (eg, axioms, propositions, laws) is not accidental. Indeed, mathematics is an ideal logistic method; its rules for interrelationships of particular variables (quantities) are highly specified, invariate, and closely bound in a unified system. Logistic theorists aspire to reduce their theories to mathematics-like formulas. Roy (1989) uses a logistic method:

The Roy Adaptation Model can be viewed primarily as a systems model though it also contains interactionist levels of analysis. The person as patient is viewed as having parts or elements linked together in such a way that force on the linkages can be increased or decreased. Increased force, or tension, comes from strains within the system or from the environment that impinges on the system. The system of the person and his interaction with the environment are thus the units of analysis of nursing assessment, while manipulation of parts of the system or the environment is the mode of nursing intervention. The person has four subsystems: physiologic needs, self-concept, role function, and interdependence. (p. 105)

In this citation Roy addresses both components of her system, which are the component parts of man and the relationships among components (eg, forces, tensions, and strains). Johnson's (1980) logistic process acts on a different subject matter (behavioral subsystems), but her method is the same:

The subsystems are linked and open, as is true in all systems, and a disturbance in one subsystem is likely to have an effect on others. . . . Although each subsystem has a specialized task or function, the system as a whole depends upon an integrated performance. (p. 210)

Johnson defines behavioral subsystems of attachment or affiliation, aggression, dependency, achievement, ingestion, elimination, and sex.

Problematic Method

The *problematic* method uses neither the parts nor some overarching whole as its basis. Instead, it acts by recognizing and defining unique problems, then reconciling the factors that constitute a given problem situation. In this sense there is a *whole* (all the constituents of the problem and its solution), but the whole is different for any given problem.

The problematic mode of thought differs from both the dialectic and logistic methods in that the problem-solver himself is part of the method, that is, he is part of the circumstance in which the problem occurs. Except for his identifying the situation as problematic, there would be nothing to initiate inquiry. This involvement of the agent in the method is quite different from the way in which dialectic and logistic methods of thought function. The structure in these other methods is independent of the agent. The component parts of Roy's hypothesized human, for example, are not altered by the agent applying her logistic method; nor does the nature of ultimate nature of consciousness change from one of Newman's nurses to another.

Reasoning in the problematic method aims at resolution through the interaction of the problem-solver and the environment. The method is the familiar one of problem-solving. Sometimes called the scientific method, problem-solving involves the following steps. The agent:

1. Interacts with the environment by means of problem encounter
2. Inquires regarding the circumstances
3. Frames hypotheses
4. Tests the implied consequences of the selected hypothesis
5. Confirms or rejects the hypothesis

In the problematic method, problems may be linked: the solution to one problem becoming the means whereby another problem is investigated. The problematic method can present an evolving chain of related problems in which ends continuously are converted to means. Such a chain, however, does not terminate in a self-sufficient and bounded system as occurs in logistic and dialectic modes of thought.

In the problematic method of thinking, each problem has its own universe, its own environment (those things that pertain to and have an impact on the problem). Problems arise only through the perception of an agent—the person who determines that a given situation is problematic. Nor is a problematic mode of thought directed toward fixed goal achievement, but rather, toward resolution of the situation (Fig. 10–3).

The problematic approach is evident in the research of Burke, Kauffmann, Costello, and Dillon (1991). They recognized a problem, when they realized that:

> . . . *disabled children not only had more hospitalizations, but also that hospitalizations were more stressful for "experienced" mothers of*

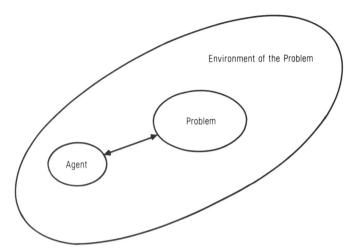

Figure 10–3.   *Pattern in problematic method.*

disabled children than for the less experienced mothers with nondisabled children. . . . The purpose of this study is to gain a better understanding of the stressful process for parents involved in repeated hospitalization of children with chronic conditions. (p. 39)

Next, the authors search the *environment* of the problem—first, unsatisfactorily, scanning available research. They find tangential reports, but nothing dealing directly with their problem, so they expand the notion of environment to include interviewing mothers of school-aged children with physical disabilities. They asked these mothers about their parental stress using a grounded theory approach. Grounded theory, incidentally, is a common method for problematic research because all the variables cannot be known at the start.

From these data three types of incidents were identified that increased stress: negative information (information that turns out to be wrong), gaps and variations in information, and inexperienced health care workers practicing on their children. Burke and coworkers summarized these as *hazardous secrets*. The parental response termed, *reluctantly taking charge,* was also found to contain three elements: vigilance and covert taking over, negotiating rules and calling a halt, and tenacious information seeking (p. 42). The problem-solving hypotheses can now be formed, for example: if hazardous secrets increase, then parental stress increases.

Levine's (1971) early work is also problematic in approach. When one examines her conservation theory, her four conservation principles are really four separate problems to be solved by the nurse for every patient: How does one conserve energy? Structural integrity?

Personal integrity? Social integrity? Levine treats each problem as its own separate universe with its own separate resolution. Unlike Roy or Johnson, Levine does not attempt to interrelate the four principles (except insofar as they all address some aspect of conservation). She does not take a logistic approach such as asking how conservation of social integrity might affect structural integrity or how conservation of energy might have an impact on personal integrity.

Nor does she weld these concepts into some dialectic synthesis of an overarching whole. *Conservation* exists only through the concrete solving of the four separate problems. Each principle is addressed singularly, unmixed with issues of the other three conservation problems. In typical problematic thinking, Levine sees each problem in its entirety, with its own resolution. Also, her system is unbounded; that is, further principles (ie, problems) may be found in the future.

One can compare Roy's (1989) concept of man with Levine's (1971) because their theory elements show some correspondence (Fig. 10–4).

Despite a superficial correspondence, there is an important difference in the two sets of elements. Roy's elements are subsystems of man, but Levine's elements are located in the nursing act. Levine's four principles compartmentalize the nursing problems, not the human being. Therefore, Levine can assert a holistic view of man. Indeed, the whole man is the subject matter for each of her discrete nursing problems.

Compare the kinds of arguments offered by Levine and Roy in support of their respective positions. Levine advances her argument by giving numerous examples of each conservation principle in action. Because problem resolution differs slightly in every situation, this sort of argument is typical of a problematic thinker. Roy, on the other hand, advances her argument by reducing each component system of man into its subcomponents: stimuli (of three sorts), adapta-

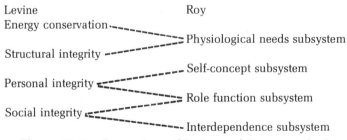

Figure 10–4.   *Comparison of Levine and Roy on method.*

tion level, and response. Relations among these more basic components are also discussed, completing the logistic linkages.

Operational Method

The *operational* method is similar to the problematic method in that the agent is part of the method. Whereas the problematic method involves an interaction between the agent and his environment, the operational method is comprised of the perspective of the agent, rather than an interaction. In a sense the agent *is* the method, and this differentiates operational from problematic thought. Method cannot be independent of the perspective and activity of the agent in operational thought. Of course, a single person may have different perspectives at different times; and there are as many methods as there are different persons to perceive and use them.

Reasoning in the operational mode is typified in debate—one perspective versus another. Selection of one viewpoint over another occurs, but it is assumed that a plurality of views will remain. The operational method moves by *discrimination* between or among points of view; it unveils differences, usually by persuasion rather than formal proof.

Selection among points of view or between courses of action is not essential in all instances of the operational method; in some circumstances, there is no need for resolution. An operational nursing theory, for example, could present alternatives among which the reader might select according to his own preferences.

Where systematic chains of reasoning occur in operational thought, movement occurs through choice among alternatives; either one perspective or another, one action or another, is chosen. *Either/or*, not synthesis, governs thought in the operational mode. Discrimination is the method used, and chains of reasoning are such that the alternative selected at the first point of choice constrains the alternatives available for choice at the second point in the chain. Whereas chains of reasoning in dialectic thought show synthesis (moving upward), a downward branching is discernible in operational thought (Fig. 10–5). At each step of operational thought, alternatives or finer and finer discriminations are identified.

In the operational method, the actions of the agent determine knowledge. For example, a foot (in length) in operational thought is not some absolute in itself; it is instead the operations of the agent that mark off a foot. An operational definition would not assert that a foot in one set of temporal-spatial coordinates is identical in length with a foot in another set of coordinates, but simply that the agent performs the same acts in each setting (ie, the foot is defined by

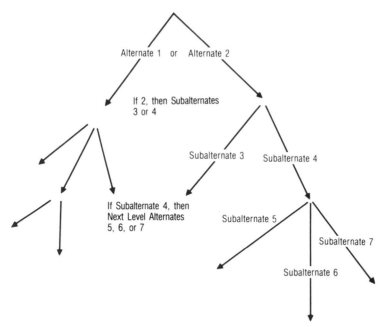

Figure 10–5. *Pattern in operational method.*

what is *done* rather than by what *is*). The methodology leading to knowledge rests in the action and the perspective of the agent.

Orem (1985, pp. 38–39) is an operational thinker. Her argument moves by telling what the agent does—what discriminations the nurse makes among patient needs, what selection she makes among all modes of care. Orem's concept of self-care is subjected to operational differentiation. Self-care (an activity) is divided on the basis of who does it: *either* the patient *or* the nurse.

In operational fashion, Orem differentiates self-care into three types: universal self-care requisites, development self-care requisites, and health-deviation self care requisites (p. 90). She further divides her major self-care categories according to specific areas in which the patient may need assistance. For universal self-care, Orem identifies eight possible loci for which the patient may require maintenance, provision, or prevention: (1) intake of air, (2) intake of water, (3) intake of food, (4) elimination processes and excrements, (5) balance between activity and rest, (6) balance between solitude and social interaction, (7) hazards to life and well-being, and (8) human functioning and developing within groups (normalcy) (pp. 90–91).

Each segment of Orem's theory shows a similar operational pattern, in other words breaking each concept into subordinate either/

or options, making multiple layers of discriminations of one sort or another. It would be possible to diagram Orem's book in an extensive series of downward branching chains of organization.

Medicine has adopted an operational method for most of its education and practice, whereas nursing has few operational theories. In medicine, the notion of *differential diagnosis* indicates the operational thought pattern. Although nursing process could be designed in an operational fashion, it is seldom so presented. Nursing process is usually given in a logistic fashion. However, nurse practitioners appear to use operational thought much like physicians when they focus on the patient's presenting symptoms.

Orlando (1990) uses operational discriminations. For example, she differentiates observations (raw material) into direct and indirect (p. 7) from which she draws consequences: to act or not to act (p. 8). Even her basic principle hinges on a difference: the nurse's interpretation of the patient's behavior versus what it meant to the patient. If one examines her writing, the discriminating and selecting can be seen to resemble the same process applied by Orem.

THE READER'S TASK

The reader is encouraged to read concurrently the theory works addressed in this chapter. This way the analyses presented here can be meaningful. Only in careful reading, rereading, and reasoned diagnosis will the reader develop the skills necessary for analyzing theories. The reader should bear in mind that: (1) a principle is a statement that is key to how a theory works, (2) an interpretation is a statement as to *what* characterizes the circumstances (ie, what reality is like); and (3) method is the characteristic manner in which an author thinks and organizes her assertions, statements, or arguments.

Not all theorists are consistent in the principles, interpretation, and method they apply. For example, a theorist may use a problematic method in one place, a logistic method in another. The best theories, however, are consistent. Confusion results if the theorist arbitrarily switches back and forth, for example, between a physiologically based explanation of man (interpretation) and an explanation of man as psychological. If the reader has trouble analyzing a given theory, she should consider that the problem may be the author's inconsistencies.

ALTERNATE MODELS

Not all critics of theory analyze principle, interpretation, and method. Chinn and Kramer (1991), for example, suggest four structural devices for analytical purposes: a triangle, a circle, a continuum, and differentiation.

> *The triangular drawing suggests that health is comprised of a series of related subconcepts that vary in breadth or simplicity. It also suggests foundational concepts upon which other subconcepts are built. (p. 116)*
>
> *The overlapping circles depict discrete components that have common areas between and among them. (p. 116)*
>
> *Applying this idea to the horizontal line drawing on the figure shows "health" represented as a continuum. This structure suggests that health is in a linear relationship with illness. (p. 117)*
>
> *The fourth structural form conveys the ideal of differentiation, dividing major concepts into subconcepts. (p. 117)*

These structures bear some relationship to the materials discussed earlier in this chapter. The triangle, with broad foundational concepts on which more narrow notions are built, is virtually the opposite of the dialectic—in which reasoning starts with the narrow and moves to the broad. The second device (illustrated by a Venn diagram of three interlocking circles) does not represent any methodology discussed here, but certainly could be interpreted as a boundary demarcation. The third device, using a continuum rather than separation of opposing aspects, is often found in transcendental, ontic interpretations. Chinn and Kramer's final structure is essentially the opposite of their triangle image and roughly equivalent to the operational method as presented in this chapter.

Chinn and Kramer are not the only good critics of theory. The reader should also peruse books by Meleis (1991), Fawcett (1993, 1995), Fitzpatrick and Whall (1996), and Walker and Avant (1995).

SUMMARY

The nurse who truly wants to understand theory needs to apply diverse analytical devices to her reading. This chapter has presented one such construct: the notion of a theory as a combination of principle, interpretation, and method. This method of analysis may be difficult for the nurse with little background in philosophy. Because it is not the only method available to her, she should not concerned if she prefers other methods.

Nevertheless, taking a theory apart as to principle, interpretation, and method, even if the analysis is imperfect, will provide the reader with insight into the theory. This exercise may be particularly valuable if a given theory appears abstruse or radically different from others she has studied.

REFERENCES

Arakelian, M. (1980, October). An assessment of nursing application of the concept of locus of control. *Advances in Nursing Science, 1,* 25–42.

Burke, S. O., Kauffmann, E., Costello, E. A., & Dillon, M. C. (1991, Spring). Hazardous secrets and reluctantly taking charge: Parenting a child with repeated hospitalizations. *Image, 1,* 39–45.

Chinn, P. L., & Kramer, M. K. (1991). *Theory and nursing: A systematic approach* (3rd ed.). St. Louis: Mosby-Year Book.

Fawcett, J. (1993). *Analysis and evaluation of nursing theories.* Philadelphia: Davis.

Fawcett, J. (1995). *Analysis and evaluation of conceptual models of nursing.* Philadelphia: Davis.

Fitzpatrick, J. J., & Whall, A. L. (1996). *Conceptual models of nursing: Analysis and application* (3rd ed.). Stamford, CT: Appleton & Lange.

Flaskerud, J. H., Halloran, E. J., Janken, J., Lund, M., & Zetterlund, J. (1979). Avoidance and distancing: A descriptive view of nursing. *Nursing Forum, 2,* 158–174.

Hall, L. E. (1966). Another view of nursing care and quality. In K. M. Straub & K. S. Parker (Eds.), *Continuity of patient care: The role of nursing* (pp. 47–66). Washington, DC: Catholic University Press.

Hardy, M. E. (1973). The nature of theories. In M. E. Hardy (Ed.), *Theoretical foundations for nursing,* New York: MSS Information Corporation.

Johnson, D. E. (1980). The behavioral system model for nursing. In J. P. Riehl & C. Roy (Eds.), *Conceptual models for nursing practice* (2nd ed., pp. 207–216). New York: Appleton-Century-Crofts.

Jones, P. A. (1978, November). An adaptation model for nursing practice. *American Journal of Nursing, 11,* 1900–1906.

King, I. M. (1981). *A theory for nursing: Systems, concepts, process.* New York: Wiley.

Levine, M. E. (1971, June). Holistic nursing. *Nursing Clinics of North America, 2,* 253–264.

McKeon, R. (n.d.). *Philosophic semantics and philosophic inquiry.* Chicago: mimeograph for University of Chicago doctoral students, 1950s.

McKeon, R. (1954). *Thought, action and passion.* Chicago: University of Chicago Press. (Concepts of principle, interpretation, and method as used in this book are taken from these organizing structures appearing in the various works of Richard McKeon.)

Meleis, A. F. (1991). *Theoretical nursing: Development and progress* (2nd ed.). Philadelphia: Lippincott.

Neuman, B. (1980). The Betty Neuman health-care systems model: A total person approach to patient problems. In J. P. Riehl & C. Roy (Eds.), *Conceptual models for nursing practice* (2nd ed., pp. 119–131). New York: Appleton-Century-Crofts.

Newman, M. A. (1994). *Health as expanding consciousness* (2nd ed.). St. Louis: Mosby.

Orem, D. E. (1985). *Nursing: Concepts of practice* (3rd. ed.). New York: McGraw-Hill.

Orlando, I. J. (1990). *The dynamic nurse-patient relationship.* New York: National League for Nursing Press.

Paterson, J. G., & Zderad, L. T. (1988). *Humanistic nursing.* New York: National League for Nursing Press.

Rogers, M. E. (1970). *An introduction to the theoretical basis of nursing.* Philadelphia: Davis.

Rogers, M. E. (1990). Nursing: Science of unitary, irreducible, human beings: Update 1990. In E. A. M. Barrett (Ed.), *Visions of Roger's science-based nursing* (pp. 1–11). New York: National League for Nursing Press.

Roy, C. (1989). The Roy adaptation model. In J. Riehl-Sisca (Ed.), *Conceptual models for nursing practice* (3rd ed., pp. 179–188). Norwalk, CT: Appleton & Lange.

Smith, J. A. (1981, April). The idea of health: A philosophical inquiry. *Advances in Nursing Science, 3,* 43–50.

Walker, L. O., & Avant, K. C. (1996). *Strategies for theory construction in nursing* (3rd ed.). Norwalk, CT: Appleton & Lange.

Watson, J. (1988). *Nursing: Human science and human care: A theory of nursing.* New York: National League for Nursing Press.

11 *The Nursing Process and Problem-Solving*

Nursing process and problem-solving theories are considered in the same chapter, not because they are alike, but because people often confuse them. In fact, their structures are quite different. This is not to deny that the two theories are intermixed in some organizations, creating an inconsistent ideology. For example, a nursing service may require problem-oriented charting while simultaneously advocating the use of the nursing process. The basic incompatibility of these theories is discussed after each theory is reviewed separately.

THE NURSING PROCESS

Often an incomplete theory evolves in the practice setting or in the nursing literature before it is recognized as a theory; this has been the case with the nursing process. Highly popular before its theory implications were fully understood, the nursing process is still not always recognized as a theory thread. Frisch (1995, p. 51), for example, argues that nursing diagnosis and theory can be combined, not realizing that nursing diagnosis is already a nursing theory component, namely, a process element. The evolution of nursing process toward full theory status has been taking place over more than three decades: first, development of the process itself; next, the addition of content elements in the form of nursing diagnoses; and now, nursing interventions as the next content piece.

The term *nursing process* has been given many different meanings. Sometimes authors change the meaning of the term without even realizing it. The nursing literature commonly talks of *the* nursing process, not *a* nursing process, as if there were only one formulation. This is far from the truth, but we will work within a flexible description.

However cast, the nursing process is a procedure for organizing nursing care that begins with patient assessment. This step leads to the second step, which cannot be initiated until information has been garnered and processed at the preceding step. This format (each step dependent on conclusions reached or acts completed in the prior step) continues through all the steps of the process until the last step (evaluation) is concluded. Often the information acquired at the final step completes a circle, starting the process again.

The content and number of steps in the nursing process account for the variability in definitions. Some formulations hold as few as four steps (assess, plan, implement care, evaluate); other formulations might have any number of the following steps:

1. Patient assessment
2. Nursing diagnosis
3. Patient prognosis
4. Goal setting
5. Therapeutic care planning
6. Care implementation
7. Evaluation of
   a. Patient status (reassessment after care)
   b. Accuracy of prior assessment
   c. Goal achievement
   d. Accuracy of prognosis
   e. Appropriateness of therapeutic choices
   f. Effectiveness of care delivery
   g. Needed alterations in the plan

Patient prognosis is omitted in many models. Similarly, evaluation often fails to consider the quality of the care implementation. In some formulations, the reassessment is conceptualized as initiating a new nursing process rather than completing an ongoing one. For this discussion, the nursing process will refer to the process depicted above, whether or not its formulation includes all the possible, logical steps.

The nursing process is logistic, having a format of discrete components related to each other in unvaried, prescribed, and inflexible sequence. For example, one never implements care before making a therapeutic plan; one never diagnoses before assessing. The nature of the process forces its user to think in terms of interrelated components. Completeness means doing all the parts.

If one were to identify the process theory thread most dominant in nursing today, the nursing process would be that thread. Its use is prevalent in the standards of care published by the American Nurses Association (ANA), and it has also been adopted in a large number of nursing schools and practice settings. When one method of practice receives such extensive adoption, one must consider that the model has much to recommend it. That is certainly the case with the nursing process. First, it somewhat resembles the medical model and can be used for professional parallelism. Simply put, it is a way to assert that the nursing profession is just as mature as medicine. Of course, Henderson's (1987) insight on the process notes that parallelism may also mean separatism and failures in collaboration.

Perhaps the greatest appeal of the nursing process is that it offers a system for uniform practice. As with other logistic systems, the nursing process is unvaried, that is, designed so that any number of nurses applying it correctly, come to the same conclusions—at least that is the ideal to be desired. In a profession seeking to be a science, this aspect of the system appeals. Because the nursing process encourages uniformity of practice, it enhances the possibilities of research, especially research applying quantitative measures. A strong commitment to this method of research on the part of many nurses helps account for the system's popularity. Extensive adoption indicates the process has perceived superiority over other formats, but there are major disagreements about its efficacy.

Another reason for the popularity of nursing process is its adaptability. As a theory thread, the nursing process is compatible with the many other logistic systems on the present health care scene (such as computer-generated management and information systems). For a generation of nurses raised on computers, the nursing process feels comfortable. It is no coincidence that many leaders most heavily committed to the nursing process are the same people actively involved in the effort to identify a minimum nursing data set (the objective of which is to allow institutions to collect uniform data) (Werley & Lang, 1988). Both systems are logistic with similar world views; both focus on nursing as a science in which nurses can replicate the judgments and research findings of their colleagues.

Because the nursing process is a *process* rather than a *content* element, it has the appeal of telling the nurse what to do. The process element is the weak link in many extant nursing theories, so it is not surprising that nurses are pleased to find a promising action directive.

Limitations

This is not to say that the nursing process has no flaws; every system has its limitations. Benner (1984) recognized an important one. Using the Dreyfus Model of Skill Acquisition (Dreyfus & Dreyfus, n.d.), she constructed a model of nursing research designed to explore clinical excellence. The Dreyfus model describes five separate levels of skill acquisition, and Benner, accordingly, differentiated nursing practice into these five levels.

The five levels are: (1) novice, (2) advanced beginner, (3) competent performer, (4) proficient performer, and (5) expert. Briefly, the levels can be characterized in the following way. The novice learns context-free rules to guide her action. She gains few subtleties in understanding; she simply applies the objectifiable rules. The advanced beginner starts to appreciate some "aspects of the situation" that require prior experience for recognition. The advanced beginner still needs help in setting priorities and sorting out what is important from what is not. She is only beginning to recognize recurrent meaningful patterns. The competent performer (a level reached after 2–3 years of practice) begins to see her actions in terms of long-range goals and plans. She lacks speed and flexibility but has a feeling of mastery and the ability to cope with many contingencies. The proficient performer sees situations as wholes rather than being concerned with isolated aspects. She recognizes when the expected picture fails to materialize and no longer relies on rules or analytical principles. The expert performer can actually be impaired by rules and principles. She has an intuitive grasp of each situation and zeroes in on problems and solutions without wasting time considering alternatives. The knowledge imbedded in practice becomes visible.

The Dreyfus educational model allowed Benner to segregate and rank anecdotes about excellent practice among nurses. An important finding was that the nursing process worked better at lower levels of expertise than at higher ones. This may account for its popularity in schools (it provides a structure for the learner) and it explains why many experienced, practicing nurses seem to ignore it.

Benner found the need for a rigidly controlled system (and the nursing process/nursing diagnosis system is that) was greatest for the novice or advanced beginner but that such high control actually impaired the work of the expert nurse. As Benner (1984) said, "If experts are made to attend to the particulars or to a formal model or rule, then performance actually deteriorates." (p. 37)

THEORY BUILDING WITH NURSING PROCESS

Alone, the nursing process is simply a theory strand, not a complete theory. The attempt to build a comprehensive theory around it can be seen in two movements: (1) the use of the nursing process in conjunction with other theories that lack a process element, and

(2) the effort to taxonomize nursing diagnoses and interventions as complementary content pieces.

Capers and Kelly (1987, p. 19) illustrate the first tactic when they append the nursing process to Neuman's theory. Neuman's theory, like the nursing process, is logistic and reductionist, so combining these two systems is possible. In the adaptation made here, the authors used Neuman's organizing categories of psychological, physiologic, developmental, sociocultural, and spiritual as the content items (diagnostic categories) to which the nursing process was applied.

One can envision a similar appending of nursing process to Johnson's content categories (human behavioral systems). One could *not* use the same tactic on Roy's theory, on the other hand, even though she has a logistic system, for she has developed her own process element (stimulus–response manipulation). The introduction of the nursing process into this work would be a major theory alteration. (Of course, some are doing just that.)

The more common tactic is not to link nursing process with an extant theory but to produce new content to accommodate it. Loomis and Wood (1983) give an example of such a constructed theory. Their process element (called clinical decision-making) is a formulation of the nursing process with elements of data collecting, diagnosing, planning, treating, and evaluating. In their model, a second set of interfacing components identifies actual or potential health problems, including: developmental life changes, acute health deviation, chronic health deviation, and cultural/environmental stressors. These theory elements can best be interpreted as *context* elements, that is, circumstances under which nursing occurs. A final set of factors identifies human responses, including physical, emotional, cognitive, familial, social, and cultural. This set represents *content* items.

The Loomis and Wood model illustrates a nursing theory constructed by combining nursing process with other elements, in this case, health problems and human responses. A more common tactic is to link nursing process with nursing diagnoses.

Nursing Diagnosis and Intervention

Although nursing diagnosis has wide acceptance in nursing, there has never been consensus on what it means. Yet the work on nursing diagnosis is one of the few successful group endeavors in theory building. Gebbie and Lavin (1975) reported on the initial 1973 work of the First National Conference on the Classification of Nursing Diagnoses. As one might expect, the first group effort produced as much confusion as light. From the start, complaints arose about many of the items labeled as diagnoses. The same year that the report was published, Gebbie (1975) clarified the definition of a nursing diagnosis in the following way:

> . . . *a nursing diagnosis is a label for a condition most clearly identified by nurses, and amenable to treatment using the range of nursing skills. It remains a nursing diagnosis even if made by another; for example, "sensory deprivation" would seem to many to be a nursing rather than a medical diagnosis. . . .*
> . . . *what is a diagnosis in one discipline may be a sign of a different diagnosis in another. For example, "fracture of femur" is a medical diagnosis. "Limitation of mobility" is accepted by many as a nursing diagnosis. (p. 69)*

The diagnoses determined by that First Nursing Conference on Classification of Nursing Diagnoses represented many different sorts of items (Gebbie & Lavin, 1974, pp. 62–112). They included:

1. States of being experienced by the patient—and possibly inferred by the nurse (eg, pain, anxiety, confusion)
2. Physiologic deviations from the norm (eg, irregular bowel function, impaired mobility)
3. Patient behaviors perceived as problematic by the nurse (eg, noncompliance, manipulation)
4. Altered relationships by the patient, on which value judgments have been placed by the nurse (eg, alteration in faith in God, altered relations with self and others)
5. Reactions of another party (eg, significant other's adjustment to patient's illness)

Work on nursing diagnosis is still underway, now carried on by individuals and in group activity by the North American Nursing Diagnosis Association (NANDA). NANDA (1989) released a taxonomy of diagnoses, probably the most used taxonomy today. Even though this group has made refinements in what constitutes a diagnosis, the taxonomy still has its critics—as does nursing diagnosis itself. Nor is the list of diagnoses out of the woods yet. Frisch (1995, p. 51), for example, claims that the introduction of the new diagnosis, energy field disturbance, permits Rogerian, holistic theories to come within the venue of the nursing process. This is a clear misunderstanding (on her part and on the part of the list makers) of clear differences in methodology between the nursing process and the methods of holistic nursing.

Porter's (1986) assertion that NANDA subordinated the task of creating a taxonomy to politics is still a cogent argument:

These purposes [for having a taxonomy] are all related to promoting the unique identity of the nursing profession; while this is a commendable aim, it is quite different from the traditional purpose of taxonomic development. (p. 136)

She reminds us that taxonomies are used to explain why an object has various properties similar to and different from others in its class. This precludes the NANDA attempts to force nursing diagnoses into a conceptual framework consisting of categories that are not mutually exclusive or jointly exhaustive.

Although Porter addresses the NANDA work in specific terms, Turkoski's (1988) concerns revolve around the nature of a nursing diagnosis, and she identifies disagreements on many poles: whether a nursing diagnosis can also be a medical diagnosis, whether a nursing diagnosis is different from a nursing assessment, and whether individual items qualify in various taxonomies.

Mitchell, Gallucci, and Fought (1991, p. 154) call for a new organization for diagnoses, suggesting the following four human responses: behavioral, experiential, pathophysiologic, and physiologic. Nor are they the only critics who would change the work being done on the diagnosis element. On the whole, disagreements are fewer these days and categories—at least those evolved by NANDA—have been refined and extended.

Just as we found authors who applied the nursing process to theories that lacked a process element, so we find authors trying to link the notion of nursing diagnosis to already existing theories. Jenny (1989) attempted to reconcile the NANDA classification with Orem's (process) concept of self-care. Because Orem's process is operational instead of logistic, it would take much revision of the nursing process to make this work.

For work on diagnosis done by individuals, see, for example, diagnostic taxonomies by Doenges and Moorhouse (1988); Gordon (1982); Kim, McFarland, and McLane (1984); and Carpenito (1997). All of these systems have taken a second seat to the NANDA work, however. Now another necessary content item, interventions, has been addressed in two taxonomies. No one is doing work on taxonomies for prognoses or goal setting, however—categories that logically fit between diagnosis and intervention. These two steps of the nursing process have never received much attention and are often hidden intellectual steps unrecognized even by the nurses who perform them.

The work of Bulechek and McCloskey (1987) heralded the beginning of serious work on the intervention phase. Their early work specified nursing interventions that were separate from physicians' orders, activities that fell within the independent role of nursing.

They included actions such as relaxation training, counseling, values clarification, music therapy, and exercise programs among others.

Their work at the University of Iowa has now grown beyond the esoteric interventions of holistic nursing into an endeavor to truly capture all the normal interventions that constitute the work of nursing. This endeavor is part of the effort to create a nursing minimum data set (Werley & Lang, 1988). The final set is envisioned as containing nursing diagnoses, interventions, and patient outcomes.

Bulechek and McCloskey (1992, p. 290) differentiate between diagnoses and interventions by saying that a diagnosis represents a client behavior or status, whereas an intervention describes a nurse behavior. Their labels consist of three words or less, such as *bleeding reduction: nasal* or *cardiac care: acute* (pp. 293–294). The created labels are extensive, with over 3,000 nursing activities considered and over 400 resultant labels (1992, p. 291), with the project still ongoing.

The second taxonomy of interventions was organized for nurses in home health care (Saba et al., 1991). Saba and colleagues developed a computerized classification system for Medicare patient services; 80,000 textual descriptions were used as a data source, making the system one of the most comprehensive data sets yet to surface.

No theory is without limitations, and that is certainly true of the nursing process/diagnosis/intervention model. Although the nursing process steps are easily learned and used by inexperienced nurses, the nursing diagnoses are so numerous as to make application a trial. The same can be said for the taxonomies of nursing interventions. The question is whether such a complex system can have a major impact on practice. Can the computer satisfactorily be substituted for the human memory in working with a theory? No matter how the system is computerized, a human must interact with it and make decisions.

The argument for the complex system of diagnoses and interventions is that a similar system of diagnostic classification has worked effectively in medicine for years. Yet there is a difference in the two applications. Physicians use an operational system (differential diagnosis) rather than a logistic schema. They feel no need to consider the whole list of possibilities; they select those that suit their purposes and deal with them alone. Nor do physicians feel a need to refer to the official codes when diagnosing and treating patients. Nurses, in contrast, view the lists of diagnoses as documents to use in relation to client work, not as a system primarily for statistical and taxonomic (as opposed to clinical) purposes.

Weber (1991), aware of the criticisms against nursing diagnosis, claims that the fault lies in the application, not in the diagnoses themselves. Geissler (1991) adds a further criticism to the work of NANDA, claiming it is culture bound when looked at from a transcultural nursing perspective. She summarizes the following flaws:

1. *Assuming the patient is "wrong" and the provider is "right"*
2. *Generalizing or stereotyping behaviors*
3. *Mislabeling the etiological basis of a patient's problem as cultural without recognizing other potentially more relevant variables (p. 203)*

Scahill (1991) voices a concern that the separate list of nursing diagnoses may put nurses at risk of isolation in multidisciplinary settings such as psychiatry. The use of NANDA diagnostic labels has always been especially tricky in psychiatry. For a sense of these complexities, see Vincent and Coler's (1990) attempt to bridge the gap between NANDA efforts and the classification work of the ANA Task Force on the Classification of Phenomena in Psychiatric-Mental Health Nursing.

Nevertheless, the system of nursing diagnosis is designed for reaching an acceptable level of agreement among users, and its final success or failure will be judged on that basis. So far the results are mixed. Levin, Krainovitch, Bahrenburg, and Mitchell (1989), for example, found that five of six tested diagnoses (NANDA list) reached acceptable levels of agreement among users. In contrast, Andersen and Briggs (1988, p. 144) found nurses lacked proficiency in formulating valid nursing diagnoses. The Dennison and Keeling (1989) study of one NANDA category, knowledge deficit, found serious problems with the concept. These are only three of many studies, and, so far, there is no consensus on content validity or reliability of the labels.

PROBLEM-ORIENTED NURSING

Like the nursing process, problem-oriented nursing is a partial theory. Alone, it lacks context, content, and goal. Just as the nursing process is commonly linked to one or another content item, so problem-oriented nursing is comprised of a method (problem-solving) that may be linked to various patient or nursing problems (content).

Problem-oriented nursing is a model that competes with the nursing process in practice. Originating with Dewey and applied early in educational theory, problem-solving was described as the problematic method in the preceding chapter. To differentiate the problem-solving structure from that of the nursing process, a brief comparison will be made:

1. Problem-solving occurs when a nurse meets an obstacle— situational or intellectual—that starts her on a search for

more information. The nursing process, on the other hand, starts with assessment simply because a person has been labeled *patient.* There is no waiting for an obstacle to appear.

2. Problem-solving is less formal than the nursing process. There is much back and forth between the problem as tentatively cast and the environment where explanations and solutions are sought. As the problem is redefined and delimited, the environment that applies to the case itself may shift. The nursing process, in contrast, follows an invariant sequence in which the diagnosis flows from the routinized assessment data, and each subsequent step follows from the preceding one. This invariable sequence has no back and forth adjustment. Diagnoses, for example, are derived from assessments; nursing prescriptions are derived from goals set.

3. Problem-solving has as its aim defining the situation. This is more important in one sense than the solution because the character of the problem will determine the arena and characteristics of the solution sought. When achieved, the right solution is the one that gets rid of the problem. Problem-solving aims to eliminate the obstacle, and there may be diverse ways to do so. The nursing process, in contrast, does not aim to get rid of anything. Instead, it sets a specific goal (eg, to have the patient walk with a four-point gait by the third week with adequate muscle strength for crutch management). Instead of seeking a resolution, the nursing process seeks to achieve one or more identified and specified goals.

4. Problem-solving is highly personal in that the nurse initiates the process because something bothers her. If she is not bothered by a situation (eg, a patient's slowed speech), then there is not a problem to be solved. The problem only exists when she recognizes it—however tentatively she may define it. The nursing process, on the other hand, is abstracted from the personal. If the rules and processes are accurately followed, any two nurses should draw the same conclusions, set the same goals, and select like interventions.

5. The solution has less importance in problem-solving because the true solution is the removal of the problem. Once the problem has been well delimited, the potential solutions suggest themselves. In the nursing process, in contrast, the "solution" takes on the characteristic of a goal

and a given solution (goal) is sought to the exclusion of other potential solutions.

Take as an illustration a comparison of how assessment might occur in the two contrasting systems. In nursing process, assessment would be complete, from head to toe—probably working from a highly structured format. The process would be applied no matter what the patient's complaints or status. In problem-solving, in contrast, the nurse would focus on the patient's problem, and the assessments performed would be those that related to the problem. For example, if the problem were a fractured metacarpal incurred in a minor accident, the nurse would be unlikely to perform a pelvic examination—and even more unlikely to tolerate a list that said she should examine "everything."

Although problem-solving was touted as *the* nursing method at one time, it was eclipsed in popularity by the nursing process (proving the futility of advocating any one method as an absolute standard). The form in which problem-solving retains some popularity is the Weed (1978) or so-called problem-oriented system of charting. It has been adapted and adopted by many institutions. In these organizations, nurses, physicians, or both chart according to the problems evinced by the patient. Often nursing notes must be categorized according to patient problems. The structure forces the nurse to think in a problem-solving modality; she cannot chart except as her efforts relate to the resolution of one or another perceived problem. Additionally, some nurse practitioner programs advocate a problem-oriented approach, with the nurse practitioner starting with the patient's presenting problem.

As with the nursing process, the content to be used in problem-oriented nursing has been the subject of much debate. In a pure problematic version, there are no constrictions as to what counts as a problem. The nurse is the one to identify the problem; its ultimate delineation is unique, dependent on her inquiry processes. Sometimes the problem-oriented system is modified by supplying the nurse with a list of "appropriate problems" from which to select. This tactic shifts the system from a problematic format to an operational or logistic one, not unlike the use of nursing diagnosis lists. Some authorities advocate a shared list of problems between medicine and nursing; others advocate a separate and distinct list of nursing problems. In any case, once the so-called problems have already been defined, prescribed, and labeled, one is no longer actually using the problem-solving method. The crux of a problematic method is determining the unique problem.

Just as advocates of nursing process debate over the proper form for nursing diagnoses, so those recommending problem-solving argue over what type of problem qualifies. Some like the perspective of *nursing* problems, that is, problems for the nurse such as fluid and electrolyte imbalance, cyanosis, failure to comply with a nursing regimen. Others select *patient* problems, such as pain anxiety or immobility, in other words, problems directly perceived by patients.

BLENDING PROBLEM-SOLVING AND THE NURSING PROCESS

Not all authors make the discrimination that this book offers between problem-solving and the nursing process. Despite that, I think mixing these modalities is confusing and makes caring for patients more difficult for nurses. Consider, for example, the nurse who must fill out a nursing care plan based on the nursing process yet simultaneously chart in accordance with a problem-oriented schema. She will have difficulty determining which modality directs her nursing behavior. McHugh (1986) offers a careful analysis of this issue from the perspective of what the nursing process is and is not.

Other authors see problem-solving and the nursing process as perfectly compatible systems. For example, LaMonica (1979) equates nursing diagnoses in one system with problems in the other. She finds other parallels between the two systems, equating both nursing process and problem-oriented recording with the scientific method (p. 318). She finds their differences more a matter of form than substance. LaMonica is not alone in this interpretation; many other nurses treat the two systems as identical.

SUMMARY

Many theory threads are used in today's practice of nursing. These threads comprise partial theories of nursing. Some are being further developed with the aim of producing a comprehensive theory. Others are conjoined with diverse theory strands, participating in many different theories (complete or partial). At present, the two most popular process threads are nursing process and problem-solving. But the nursing process far exceeds problem-oriented nursing in popularity.

REFERENCES

Andersen, J. E., & Briggs, L. L. (1988, Fall). Nursing diagnosis: A study of quality and supportive evidence. *Image, 3*, 141–144.

Benner, P. (1984). *From novice to expert: Excellence and power in clinical nursing practice.* Menlo Park, CA: Addison-Wesley.

Bulechek, G. M., & McCloskey, J. C. (1987, May). Nursing interventions: What they are and how to choose them. *Holistic Nursing Practice, 3,* 36–44.

Bulechek, G. M., & McCloskey, J. C. (1992, June). Defining and validating nursing intervention. *Nursing Clinics of North America, 2,* 289–299.

Capers, C. F., & Kelly, R. (1987, May). Neuman nursing process: A model of holistic care. *Holistic Nursing Practice, 3,* 19–26.

Carpenito, L. J. (1997). *Handbook of nursing diagnosis* (7th ed.). Philadelphia: Lippincott.

Dennison, P. D., & Keeling, A. W. (1989, Fall). Clinical support for eliminating the nursing diagnosis of knowledge deficit. *Image, 3,* 142–144.

Doenges, M. E., & Moorhouse, M. F. (1988). *Nurse's pocket guide: Nursing diagnosis with interventions* (2nd ed.). Philadelphia: Davis.

Dreyfus, S. E., & Dreyfus, H. L. (n.d.). *A five-stage model of the mental activities involved in directed skill acquisition.* Unpublished report. United States Air Force Office of Scientific Research (Contract F49620-79-C-0063), University of California at Berkeley.

Frisch, N. (1995, April/June). Nursing diagnosis and nursing theory—What does it really mean to combine the two? *Nursing Diagnosis, 2,* 51.

Gebbie, K. M. (1975). Development of a taxonomy of nursing diagnosis. In J. B. Walter, G. P. Pardee, & D. M. Molbo (Eds.), *Dynamics of problem oriented approaches: Patient care and documentation* (pp. 65–76). New York: Lippincott.

Gebbie, K. M., & Lavin, M. A. (Eds.). (1975). *Classification of nursing diagnoses.* St. Louis: Mosby.

Geissler, E. M. (1991, April). Transcultural nursing and nursing diagnoses. *Nursing & Health Care, 4,* 109–192, 203.

Gordon, M. (1982). *Manual of nursing diagnosis.* New York: McGraw-Hill.

Henderson, V. (1987, May). Nursing process—a critique. *Holistic Nursing Practice, 3,* 7–18.

Jenny, J. (1989, February). Classifying nursing diagnoses: A self-care approach. *Nursing & Health Care, 2,* 83–88.

Kim, M. J., McFarland, G. K., & McLane, A. M. (Eds.). (1984). *Pocket guide to nursing diagnoses.* St. Louis: Mosby.

LaMonica, E. L. (1979). *The nursing process: A humanistic approach.* Menlo Park, CA: Addison-Wesley.

Levin, R. F., Krainovitch, B. C., Bahrenburg, E., & Mitchell, C. A. (1989, Spring). Diagnostic content validity of nursing diagnosis. *Image, 1,* 40–44.

Loomis, M. E., & Wood, D. J. (1983, Winter). Cure: The potential outcome of nursing care. *Image, 2,* 4–7.

McHugh, M. (1986, November). Nursing process: Musings on the method. *Holistic Nursing Practice, 1,* 21–28.

Mitchell, P. H., Gallucci, B., & Fought, S. G. (1991, July/August). Perspectives on human response to health and illness. *Nursing Outlook, 4,* 154–157.

North American Nursing Diagnosis Association. (1989). *Taxonomy I revised—1989: With official diagnostic categories.* St. Louis: Author.

Porter, E. J. (1986, Winter). Critical analysis of NANDA nursing diagnosis taxonomy I. *Image, 4,* 136–139.

Saba, V. K., O'Hare, P. A., Zuckerman, A. E., Boondas, J., Levine, E., & Oatway, D. M. (1991, June). A nursing intervention taxonomy for home health care. *Nursing & Health Care, 6,* 296–299.

Scahill, L. (1991, Summer). Nursing diagnosis vs goal-oriented treatment planning in inpatient child psychiatry. *Image, 2,* 95–97.

Turkoski, B. B. (1988, May/June). Nursing diagnosis in print, 1950–1985. *Nursing Outlook, 4,* 142–144.

Vincent, K. G., & Coler, M. S. (1990, Spring). A unified nursing diagnostic model. *Image, 2,* 93–95.

Weed, L. (1978). *Medical records, medical education, and patient care.* Cleveland: Press of Case Western Reserve University.

Weber, G. (1991, October). Making nursing diagnosis work for you and your client: A step-by-step approach. *Nursing & Health Care, 8,* 424–430.

Werley, H. H., & Lang, N. M. (Eds.). (1988). *Identification of the nursing minimum data set.* New York: Springer.

BIBLIOGRAPHY

Gordon, M. (1987). *Nursing diagnosis: Process and application* (2nd ed.). New York: McGraw-Hill.

Kobert, L., & Folan, M. (1990, June). Coming of age in nursing: Rethinking the philosophies behind holism and nursing process. *Nursing & Health Care, 6,* 308–312.

12 *Systems Models in Nursing Theory*

SYSTEMS VERSUS SYSTEMATIC

Many nurse theorists claim to have a systems approach to nursing theory. In fact, some do and some do not. It is important to understand what writers mean by *systems* because different writers mean different things. For some, the meaning may be so casual as to mean systematic. Indeed, we assume that a good theory in any format would be systematic rather than chaotic. Therefore, to use the term *systems* in this fashion trivializes it.

For our purposes, we will use the term *systems model* to apply to a theory that treats its subject matter as consisting of component parts and their interrelationships. In the systems approach the focus is on the discrete parts and their interrelationships, which make up and describe the whole (ie, the system). The system (the whole) is no more than the sum of its parts and their relationships.

If this sounds familiar, it is because a logistic pattern of thought is the backbone of a systems model. Systems, then, are tightly structured designs with intentional application of logistic patterns of thought. Systems models are those in which the pattern of relationships among parts is highly prescribed. The nursing process would qualify as a systems model; the problem-solving model would not.

The subject matter addressed by a theory is not what characterizes a system. The subject matters of nursing systems include man as a system (Johnson, 1980; Neuman, 1980, 1989; Roy, 1989), the patient–nurse interaction system (King, 1981), larger systems such as communities or societies (King, 1981), and even organizations such as health care systems (Arndt & Huckabay, 1975).

For any given subject matter (eg, man as a system), there can be major differences among theorists. The components of Johnson's man–system are behavioral subsystems (such as aggression, affiliation, achievement), whereas Roy's components of the man–system are adaptation modes: physiologic, self-concept, role function, and interdependence relations. One cannot assume that the subject matter alone is a clue as to whether or not a theory is a systems model.

METHODOLOGY

Whatever their subject matter, systems-oriented theorists discuss their subject matter in ways that:

1. Differentiate the *system* from its environment (ie, identify boundary lines or events)
2. Describe input from the environment into the system as well as output from the system back to the environment (this is true for nursing models because they are open systems as opposed to a closed systems that does not interact across boundaries)
3. Identify the energy or motivation of the system (ie, what makes the system work, keep going, or, in its absence, slow down and stop)
4. Consider system equilibrium, or what keeps the system in balance, stable, within acceptable limits (as opposed to developmental changes in which the subject matter changes, evolves, takes on new goals, or radically alters its structures)
5. Identify the goals toward which the system strives and that dictate the nature of what happens in the system
6. Describe (or hope to describe) the thruput or central processing (what the system does to the input), usually in terms of a finite series of sequential acts or events over time
7. Identify feedback or cybernetic components, allowing output and goal to be compared, and giving information that is used in system adjustment
8. Explain the given system as consisting of smaller subsystems or explain the system as itself being a subsystem of a larger system

Different theorists may stress different aspects of the systems approach, while still maintaining the general design. For example, one theorist may focus on the system–environment boundary events (eg, human response to environmental stressors); another may focus on the specific nature of the thruput (structure of the central processing). A third theorist may focus on the process or movement of raw materials (input) through the system to their output as finished product, and a fourth theorist may focus on cybernetic events (eg, system adjustments in light of output).

Theories Stressing Boundary Events

Theories stressing boundary events focus on intake or exchange. For example, if man is the system under consideration, one might focus on biologic intake (food, oxygen, microbes) or on biologic exchange (the human ecology approach). The same exchange approach might be used in relation to the social environment to examine reciprocal or unequal exchanges of affect. Some ecofeminist theories are coined in terms of social exchange.

Instead of looking at the content of the materials entering or leaving the system, some theories are concerned primarily with the energy flow. Man, for example, may be seen as taking more energy from the environment than he returns to it, using the energy for growth (negentrophy). A theory such as this might use the term energy, such as Newman (1994) and Rogers (1990, 1994), but this does not mean that their theories are systems models. In fact, they are not; they are developmental models with dialectic thought structures.

Other systems theories are concerned with entry criteria. For example, do all patients constitute system input or only patients with no prior admissions for the specified condition? Good systems models are clear and crisp about their components. In this example, precise decision rules would determine what patients would qualify for processing in the system.

Theories Stressing the Structure of the Thruput

The theorist who focuses on the thruput examines the system from the perspective of structure. Thruput often is reflected in flow charts such as Figure 12-1. Such a chart shows what happens to the materials entering the system. The thruput segment is sometimes called the black box if its processes are not fully understood. In Johnson's theory, for example, the specific relationships among her subsystems of behavior are yet to be explored and described. The exact relationship of achievement behavior to affiliative behavior, for example, is

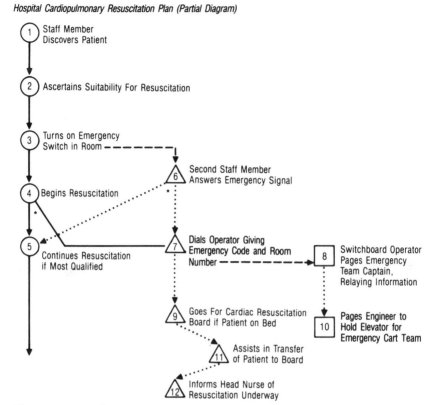

Hospital Cardiopulmonary Resuscitation Plan (Partial Diagram)

Figure 12–1. *Thruput component of a systems model, using flow charts to illustrate partial hospital cardiopulmonary resuscitation plan. *, path choice point.*

not specified. Yet, in principle, she acknowledges that these interactions of subcomponents occur.

Theories Stressing Processes of the System

The theorist who focuses on process rather than structure is likely to use a model such as Figure 12-2. Applying this model to the patient as input, one arrives at Figure 12-3. Note that in this example, the nursing organization, rather than the patient, is the system. The process traces the input from its entry from the environment to its exit back to the environment.

Theories Stressing Cybernetics

A focus on the cybernetic system concentrates on the feedback loop as illustrated in Figure 12-4. The feedback loop has three functions:

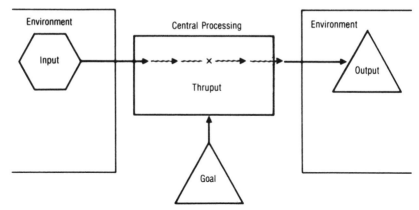

Figure 12–2. *Basic systems model (process type).*

production of data concerning system output, comparison of data to preestablished goals, and adjustment of the system for better goal achievement. Typically, the adjustment occurs in the thruput, but regulation is sometimes accomplished through change in input or alteration of the goals themselves. For example, if 5% of patients in a given nursing home developed decubitus ulcers when the goal stated less than 1%, three possibilities exist for producing conformity. First, the nursing processes (thruput) could be improved. Alternately, the goal might be deemed unrealistic and raised to 5%. Finally, they might determine that most patients spoiling their record entered with decubitus ulcers already formed, and they might quit admitting patients with unhealed decubitus ulcers (changed input).

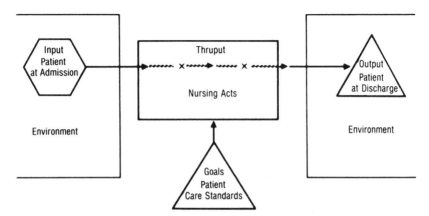

Figure 12–3. *Basic systems model of nursing care delivery.*

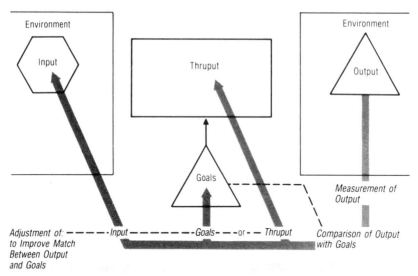

Figure 12–4. *Cybernetic loop of a systems model.*

A specific nursing goal and its measurement are illustrated in Figure 12-5. In this example, the cybernetic loop becomes the model for quality control of patient care. Patient outcomes are compared to patient care standards, and related nursing acts (thruput) will be adjusted accordingly. The Joint Commission on the Accreditation of Healthcare Organizations once focused on input (structure) and process, but now is mostly concerned with the cybernetic loop, namely, with output. This makes sense because outcomes are the whole point of health care.

MISLEADING USES OF SYSTEMS TERMINOLOGY

The confusing use of the term *systems* to cover every instance of systematic thought has been discussed. A second common error is the application of the systems label to dialectic constructs in which the whole is not only more than the sum of its parts, but gives meaning to the parts. For example, if one were to describe a nursing service organization (subject matter) as having a certain organizational *personality*, and furthermore, if one stated that this organizational personality caused head nurses to act in a particular way, then one is *not* talking in terms of a logistic system. In this example, the "system" is dialectic because characteristics of the whole (the organization) account for characteristics of the part (the head nurses).

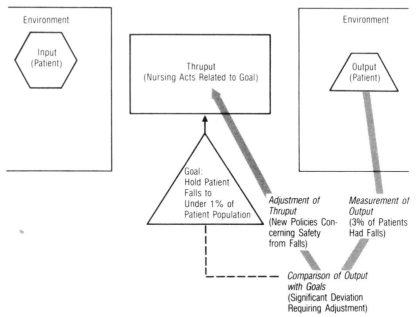

Figure 12–5. *Cybernetic loop for control of patient falls.*

A dialectic model focuses on the constellation created by the parts, not on the parts themselves. When a part is singled out for attention, it is explained by virtue of the constellation, that is, what happens to the part occurs because of its relation to the whole. A person filling the scapegoat role in a family is an example of a part (person) explained in relation to the whole (family), not in terms of that person's discrete and separate relations with other individuals in the family.

It is not unusual to see theories misclassified in nursing texts. For example, in Riehl and Roy's (1980, 2nd ed.) edited work, Rogers's theory is inappropriately listed as a systems model (corrected by Riehl-Sisca, 1989, 3rd ed.). Rogers's theory is clearly dialectic, not logistic.

Many authors differentiate logistic and dialectic models into systems and developmental models, respectively. Developmental models differ from systems models in that their goals, components, and structures are capable of and predisposed to change, usually toward ever greater levels of complexity, with qualitative changes in nature, not merely quantitative addition of new parts. Where Maslow's (1954) hierarchy of needs is seen as describing emerging stages of man, then emergence of a qualitatively different need would be developmental, an instance in which the entity itself was changed radically.

A systems model typically does not evolve and develop, but it can grow more complex by adding new components. When a new component is added, it is simply integrated with the system components already described.

Because many dialectic models also are developmental, the division between systems models and developmental models usually differentiates logistic and dialectic systems. Chrisman and Riehl-Sisca systems-developmental-stress (SDS) model (1989), however, confounds the difference between systems and developmental models, viewing man developmentally from birth to death, but claiming that in any given slice of time, he can be viewed as consisting of interlocking biologic, social, and personal systems. The system also has elements of another method, problem-solving:

> *The process, on the other hand, refers to stress and provides an approach for analyzing human problems within the structure. The patient problems that are identified can be explored and can suggest definitive implications for nursing intervention. (p. 279)*

Although verbal support is given to the developmental aspect, the SDS theory itself operates on a logistic method. As with many logistic models that take man as the subject matter, this model's input is a set of stressors, and its focus is the cybernetic adaptation of the system. Chrisman and Riehl-Sisca are aware that they are mixing methods:

> *The framework of this model incorporates aspects of human beings in the form of systems and developmental theory. Although both concepts are congruent with reality, both are required: one is not a real description of life without the other. For the purposes of analyzing human problems, the person can be conceptualized as a system moving through time and developmental stages. (p. 278)*

A third misleading use of systems terms occurs when an entity is described by a systems model (as parts and relationships), but its components and relationships do not really represent thruput processes. Take, for example, Arndt and Huckabay's (1975) model of nursing administration. Within what is claimed to be a systems model, their peculiar pattern of components and relationships is illustrated in Figure 12-6.

Diagrams and flow charts are useful to indicate relations in a systems model, but the Arndt and Huckabay diagram does not really represent a sequential flow of events. Component B is an output term, Component C is a goal term, Component D is a thruput step, and Component E probably is a side effect. The two-directional arrows of this model further confuse because, for all intents and purposes,

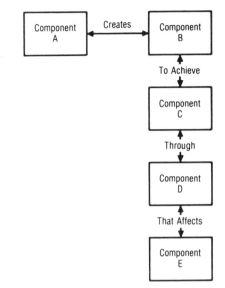

Figure 12–6.   *Segment of structural relationships, based on model by Arndt and Huckabay.*

they eliminate sequence. For example, that Component A creates Component B would seem to contradict that Component B creates A, a statement one can make equally well according to the arrows in this diagram. Although co-creation is no problem in a developmental model—see Parse (1981), for example—it just does not fit in a systems model. Hence, one distraction in analyzing theory is the application of systems-like flow charts to components and relationships that actually do not express a system.

In contrast, the systems model of the nursing process in Gordon's (1982) book—see her inside front cover—is an accurate use of systems, with each step leading the next. Gordon has elaborated 14 direct steps, formalizing some of the actions that occur unrecognized in shorter versions of the nursing process. In addition, her model has interim decision exit points (a perfectly legitimate logistic tactic) and a feedback loop.

A final problem in systems models is the overly complex model that specifies components and relationships too numerous to conceptualize. The net result of such specificity is that the reader is unable to calculate the effect of a given system manipulation. Neuman's (1980) model, interrelating over 35 variables, typifies this pattern of complexity. Although such a model may be a legitimate logistic method, it fails the test for parsimony. This is a flaw in the elaborate nursing process/diagnosis/intervention model (if it is to be used in practice rather than for computerized manipulations). Some systems have been programmed so that computers can calculate effects of system manipulations with too many variables for the human mind to simultaneously consider. For theories with massive numbers of computerized components, the best one can hope for is to intuitively grasp the principle by which the system functions.

COMPUTERIZATION AND SYSTEMS MODELS

Today much of the major growth in nursing involves the development of what is termed nursing informatics, namely, the growth and expansion in use of computerization in nursing. In addition to systems of patient diagnosis and nursing interventions, informatics include management systems that do everything from track budget variance, to calculate staffing patterns, to determine patient acuity ratings. The ways in which computers are applied to nursing will help shape tomorrow's nursing theories. Already the Internet is a great source of nursing learning and communication. Yet computers, by necessity, function in patterns of logistic (linear) relationships or in branching logic (an operational variation). It is ironic that these systems are developing side by side with holistic theories antithetical to this mode of thought.

Theories developing in the systems design today are likely to rely heavily on computer technology. True, there is some talk of computers so sophisticated that they can escape their highly prescribed program formats—a computer designed to enhance its own learning potential, for example. But it will be a long time before computers can replicate the sort of developmental, qualitative changes that are possible in holistic nursing theory.

SUMMARY

The use of systems terminology in relation to nursing theories requires close scrutiny. Writers mean different things by the term system. It would be simpler if the systems label were reserved for logistic systems to avoid this confusion. Several misleading uses of systems have been identified as consonant with this description:

1. The use of systems to describe *any* systematic work
2. The use of systems to describe dialectic or developmental constellations
3. The application of flow charts and diagrams that inaccurately appear to be logistic to describe nonlogistic theories

Even a legitimate systems model may be problematic in directing nursing practice if its variables are too numerous to grasp easily in the mind. On the other hand, good systems models, with their clear steps and controlled sequencing, are good learning tools for students and they allow for design of clear, precise research projects. The systems model also fosters the development of convenient software self-learning packages. At present, the strongest and most popular systems theory is the nursing process/diagnosis/intervention system.

REFERENCES

Arndt, C., & Huckabay, L. M. D. (1975). *Nursing administration—Theory for practice with a systems approach.* St. Louis: Mosby.

Chrisman, M. K., & Riehl-Sisca, J. D. (1989). The systems-developmental-stress model. In J. Riehl-Sisca. (Ed.), *Conceptual models for nursing practice* (3rd ed., pp. 277–295). Norwalk, CT: Appleton & Lange.

Gordon, M. (1982). *Nursing diagnosis: Process and application.* New York: McGraw-Hill.

Johnson, D. E. (1980). The behavioral system model for nursing. In J. P. Riehl & C. Roy (Eds.), *Conceptual models for nursing practice* (2nd ed., pp. 207–216). New York: Appleton-Century-Crofts.

King, I. M. (1981). *A theory for nursing: Systems, concepts, process.* New York: Wiley.

Maslow, A. H. (1954). *Motivation and personality.* New York: Harper & Row.

Neuman, B. (1980). The Betty Neuman health-care systems model: A total person approach to patient problems. In J. P. Riehl & C. Roy (Eds.), *Conceptual models for nursing practice* (2nd ed., pp. 119–134). New York: Appleton-Century-Crofts.

Neuman, B. (1989). The Neuman nursing process format: Family case study. In J. Riehl-Sisca (Ed.), *Conceptual models for nursing practice* (3rd ed., pp. 49–62). Norwalk, CT: Appleton & Lange.

Newman, M. (1994). *Health as expanding consciousness.* New York: National League for Nursing Press.

Parse, R. R. (1981). *Man-living-health: A theory of nursing.* New York: Wiley.

Riehl, J. P., & Roy, C. (1980). *Conceptual models for nursing practice* (2nd ed., pp. 329–337). New York: Appleton-Century-Crofts.

Riehl-Sisca, J. *Conceptual models for nursing practice* (3rd ed., 181–188). Norwalk, CT: Appleton & Lange.

Rogers, M. E. (1990). Nursing: Science of unitary, irreducible, human beings: Update 1990. In E. A. M. Barrett (Ed.), *Visions of Rogers' science-based nursing* (pp. 5–11). New York: National League for Nursing Press.

Rogers, M. E. (1994). Nursing science evolves. In M. Madrid & E. A. M. Barrett (Eds.), *Rogers' scientific art of nursing practice*, (pp. 3–9). New York: National League for Nursing Press.

Roy, C. (1989). The Roy adaptation model. In J. Riehl-Sisca (Ed.), *Conceptual models for nursing practice* (3rd ed., pp. 105–114). Norwalk, CT: Appleton & Lange.

13 *Criteria for Evaluating Theories*

THE NATURE OF JUDGMENT

Once a theory has been analyzed and classified, the task of passing judgment on it remains. People often view the task of judgment from one of two positions:

1. Judgment is simply a matter of personal taste. Just as some persons prefer modern art to Renaissance art, some will prefer one theory to another. The merits of a given theory ultimately are matters of personal preference and taste.
2. There are certain clear criteria for judging nursing theories. Any reasonably intelligent and informed persons, when applying these criteria, will arrive at similar judgments. Various theories are good, mediocre, or poor, and it is not only possible but reasonable to pass judgment on them.

Each position has some merit because there are some evaluative criteria on which there is little consensus and others for which consensus is strong. Few nurses, for example, would debate the criterion of consistency, which calls for the use of terms in the same way throughout a theory. Yet, there is little consensus on the criterion of scope. Some nurses judge a theory good if it covers a broad expanse of nursing practice and poor if its scope is a narrow slice of the nursing domain. Others would argue the opposite case. This chapter looks at criteria of two sorts: those receiving general acceptance and those for which no consensus exists.

Judgment of theories can be facilitated if internal and external criticisms are differentiated. Internal criticism deals with how theory components fit with each other. It asks: Given the premises this theory assumes, does the reasoning logically follow? Do the theory pieces relate in a sensible pattern? Most people agree on judgments made using criteria for internal criticism; most members of a society use similar patterns of judgment regarding what are or are not logical relations.

External criticism deals with the way in which a theory relates to the extant world. It examines the premises a theory takes as the beginning points for its propositions (ie, what is true about the world and nursing's function in it). Judgment here is highly dependent on individual preference—whether the given theory's view seems reasonable and reflects the world as perceived by the reader.

INTERNAL CRITICISM

Many criteria are applied in judging the internal construction of a theory—specifically, clarity, consistency, adequacy, and logical development. Usually there is agreement on the judgments made concerning these criteria. There is less agreement on the importance of a final criterion—the level of theory development.

Clarity

The criterion of clarity requires that a theory be presented in a way that can be best understood by the reader. The issue of clarity is not to be confused with that of the simplicity or complexity of theory development. Nor is it to be confused with the sequence in which the author presented material. The question is: Does it make sense?

In judging clarity, two sorts of meaning are given to terms. *Denotative* meaning is referential; it enables one to point out all the objects of a class, that is, all the objects to which a term refers. *Connotative* meaning indicates what denoted objects have in common. Connotation describes the characteristics of an object, giving the nuances of meaning and relaying the value bestowed.

Few authors have perfect clarity. Every author will slip now and then into a confusing sentence. But how many sentences are meaningless? Do they preclude one's understanding of the theory? Are the basic terms themselves unclear? Are the terms clear as to both denotation and connotation? Are there obvious gaps in the theory that prevent parts from linking with the subsequent aspects?

Consistency

The criterion of consistency can be applied in many different ways. We will examine inconsistencies in: terms, interpretation, principle, and method. The simplest case involves definition of terms. Once a theorist has defined a term in a certain way, consistency requires that the term always be used in that way. Common errors occur when the theorist defines:

1. Nursing—as care of individuals or groups, but then goes on to discuss it only as it applies to care of the individual
2. Stress—as a vector acting on the body, but later includes bodily responses to the vector, thus combining cause and effect (what some would call stress and strain)
3. Time—as the serial progression of clock minutes at one place and the perception of the time (the experience of duration) at another
4. Adaptation—as stimulus–response patterning, and later to mean psychological adjustment to a complex environmental change conceptualized in a Gestalt framework

The last example represents more than a simple shift in the meaning of a term. Here the fault includes a shift in the nature of the world being described. This shift in *interpretation* is a frequent fault in nursing theories. At one moment a theory may view the world as consisting of physical entities that respond on the basis of neurohumoral rules, yet in the next instance, switch to a world view in which the major entities are, instead, noncorporeal constructs, such as spheres of influence, states of mind, or phases of development. The error here does not relate to which is the *correct* interpretation of the external world (that would be an external criticism) but simply to the failure to be consistent in a world view.

Often the author does not describe the world to which the theory applies. Then the shift in the image of the world may be masked if the same theory terms are used throughout. For example, the continuous use of terms such as adaptation and stress may conceal the inconsistency of the world view. One moment adaptation may refer to responses and stimuli, the next to free will choices. Such inconsistencies in interpretation often occur in theories that purport to synthesize elements from various disparate theory statements.

In addition to finding inconsistencies in the use of terms and in interpretation, there may be inconsistencies in principle. Suppose a theory has reciprocal principles, one in the patient and one in the nursing act. Imagine that the principle explaining the patient is comprehensive (eg, explaining man as some sort of holistic being). Suppose, on the other hand, that the principle motivating the nurse is entitative, relying on a stimulus–response explanation of the nurse's behavior. Two such diverse principles would be inconsistent in a single theory; there is no logical way for the patient and nurse to inter-relate.

Similarly, one may find inconsistencies in relation to method. Sometimes this occurs when trends in nursing dictate one method, whereas the author's own inclination follows a different path. The author may use one method (her own) while giving lip service to another. In other cases, there may be fluctuations in method.

Adequacy

A theory is adequate if it accounts for the subject matter with which it purports to deal, however broad or limited. A nursing theory is adequate if its prescriptions are extensive enough to cover the scope claimed by its author.

Rubin (1968) presents an interesting theory of clinical nursing in which nursing is a helping technique "whereby the patient adjusts to, endures through, and usefully integrates the health problem situation in its many ramifications" (p. 210). In her conception, nursing care occurs in an ever-changing interaction process, dependent on the moment-to-moment situation of the patient and his ability to cope with that situation. Situations, necessarily, are fluid in this model, and nursing is differentiated from other helping professions by its operation within the immediate present in relation to the patient's dependency needs.

Some critics argue that this theory is appropriate for obstetrics (Rubin's specialty) but not for clinical nursing in general. The focus on immediacy, so say her critics, is built on the image of the patient in labor or in the midst of a major, immediate life change. The model, critics argue, fails to consider such elements as forward-looking health education or care of a patient with a chronic disease. Those who support the extended application of the theory claim that all notions of clinical nursing can be dealt with inside the model.

In some instances, a theory may so fit or misfit its purported scope that critics can easily agree on whether it meets the criterion of adequacy. In other cases, such as Rubin's, the determination of match between theory and scope may call into question the reviewer's own conception of nursing. Hence, the criterion of adequacy sometimes reflects internal criticism, and other times, branches into external criticism.

Logical Development

The criterion of logical development requires that every conclusion set forth in a theory logically follow from the reasoning that has preceded it. Logical development demands that a conclusion be warranted, based on its premises. The study of logic reveals the structure of supported and unsupported arguments. Two examples are given here, followed by the syllogistic form of each argument and an illustrative Venn diagram. These examples represent a deductive mode of reasoning in which a conclusion necessarily follows from its premises. Another mode of logical reasoning (induction) is discussed later.

In Figure 13-1, the syllogistic form of the argument goes like this:

All nursing is a form of interaction.
All communication is a form of interaction.
All nursing is a form of communication.

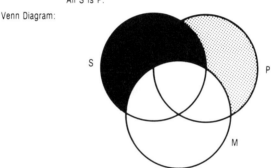

Premises: All Nursing is a Form of Interaction.
           All Communication is a Form of Interaction.
Conclusion: All Nursing is a Form of Communication.

Syllogistic All S is M.
Form: All P is M.
             All S is P.

Venn Diagram:

Figure 13–1. *Example of a deductive argument.*

Next one substitutes letters for terms, making the structure of the argument and its conclusion evident. The accompanying Venn diagram represents the interrelationship of the three terms of the argument. In the diagram, one blackens those portions of the representative circles not contained in the premises. Hence, because "All S is M" in this example, one blacks out the two segments of S that fall outside M. In looking at the second premise, two segments of P are similarly blackened. The remaining portions of the diagram reveal the error in the conclusion drawn. All remaining S is *not* P, so the argument is invalid.

Although the conclusion in the given example is patently illogical, the same pattern, given different terms, might lead one astray. Suppose, for example, that one substitutes *helping profession* for *communication.* The following argument results:

All nursing is a form of interaction.
All helping professions are forms of interaction.
All nursing is a helping profession.

The truth of the conclusion in this case might lead one astray, but it has nothing to do with the logical development of the argument. In this example, it may well be true that nursing is a helping profession, but that conclusion cannot be drawn on the basis of these premises, even if the premises were assumed to be true. Logical development has to do with whether or not conclusions can be derived from given premises, not whether or not the given premises or conclusions are true.

The next example has a slightly different format:

All protective body responses work toward establishment of
    homeostasis.
Some pain is a protective body response.
Some pain works toward establishment of homeostasis.

In Figure 13-2, the Venn diagram first blackens the inapplicable portions of the model. In addition, the second premise states that some portion of S must be M. An X is inserted in the unblackened segment that meets this constraint, indicating that some of this segment *must* exist. For this particular case, the syllogistic form can be supported (valid) because an extant segment of S falls within P, matching the conclusion drawn.

Premises: All Protective Body Responses Work Toward
                Establishment of Homeostasis.
                Some Pain is a Protective Body Response.
Conclusion: Some Pain Works Toward Establishment of Homeostasis.

Syllogistic   All M is P.
Form: Some S is M.
                Some S is P.

Venn Diagram:

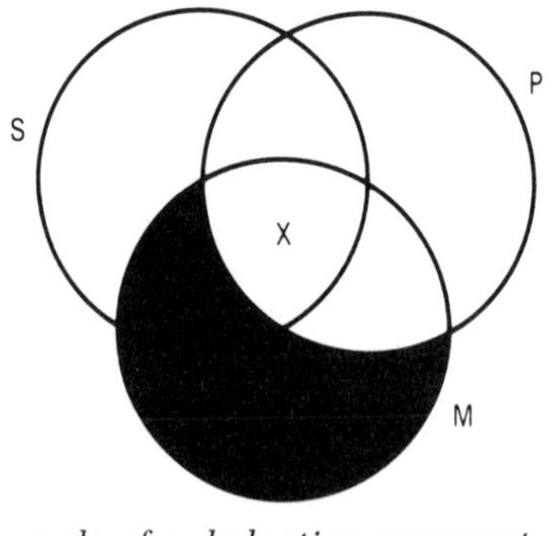

Figure 13–2. Example of a deductive argument.

Many different forms of deductive argument can be postulated, and the Venn diagram is the traditional tool for determining the valid and invalid forms. In a deductive argument, one can say that a valid form is one in which the conclusion necessarily follows from the given premises, and further, that if the premises were true, then the conclusion necessarily is true.

Inductive argument, in contrast, is based on probability rather than necessity. Induction depends on cases known, and the probability factor can always be changed by new, and contrary, cases. A typical inductive argument follows:

Morphine is a narcotic and relieves pain.
Codeine is a narcotic and relieves pain.
Heroin is a narcotic and relieves pain.
Therefore all narcotics relieve pain.

This inductive argument proves to be false because some narcotics do not relieve pain. A single exception is all that is required to invalidate an inductive conclusion when the argument deals with absolutes. (It only takes one black swan to invalidate the assertion that all swans are white.) In the so-called soft sciences, inductive patterns may be tempered by frequency qualifiers or probability hedges (eg, *most* patients prefer to know their diagnosis).

The logical development of an argument to its conclusions should not be confused with the sequence used by the author in the written presentation. It is possible that the author may: (1) present the premises first, drawing the conclusions subsequently, or (2) reveal the conclusions first, followed by the premises and argument from which they were derived. Logical development of a theory refers to the validity of its arguments, not to the sequence in the written presentation.

Logical development requires that a reader not have to supply missing links in an argument to get to the author's conclusion. Often the reader unconsciously supplies missing links, relying on her professional knowledge rather than on the theory as outlined. Indeed, the nurse may be unaware that she is filling in gaps.

Some of the logical steps in the nursing process, for example, often are missing in written formulations. Take prognosis, for example; it influences nursing action in ways the nurse seldom thinks about. Imagine a patient with a severed spinal cord above the waist. Without recognizing that she is making a prognosis, the nurse will arrange her care around the thought that the patient will not walk again. (This, of course, precludes some of the interesting new electronic/computerized systems that provide an external stimulus to replace cord function allowing a mechanized walk.)

The criterion of logical development, then, requires that a theory grow naturally from its premises, that its propositions follow from application of the rules of logic, and that any assertion or conclusion drawn flows reasonably from the groundwork laid for the assertion.

Level of Theory Development

The ultimate aim of any theory is to reach the stage in which purposeful nursing interventions can be derived, leading to predictable patient outcomes—in other words, an explanatory theory with situation-producing capabilities. The level of theory development, however, is a function of historical time; every theory, at one time, begins with the descriptive naming of its elements.

It is possible that one theory, still in a descriptive phase, may hold more promise than another theory already in an explanatory phase of development. Therefore, a relatively low (early) level of theory development is not necessarily a black mark, not in the same sense that lack of clarity, lack of consistency, or lack of logical development would be. Assessment of the level of theory development is an essential part of internal criticism.

EXTERNAL CRITICISM

External criticism evaluates a nursing theory as it relates to the real world of man, nursing, and health. In external criticism, critics generally agree that the following criteria should be achieved: reality convergence, utility, significance, and capacity for discrimination. However, there may be differences concerning whether or not a theory successfully achieves a given criterion. There is little consensus on two other criteria: scope and complexity. Critics take various stances on these criteria, favoring greater or lesser scope, more or less complexity.

Reality Convergence

Reality convergence is considered as it relates to principle, interpretation, and method. A theory may veer significantly from the real world in one or more of these aspects. Every theory is built on one or more essential principles. Principles are the crucial premises of a theory. As a theory develops, the conclusions of earlier arguments often become the premises in later assertions, thus creating linked chains of reasoning. Nevertheless, every argument starts somewhere, with a set of premises that is not supported by prior argument. It is these premises that determine the reality convergence of the theory as to principle. Whether the original premises are the principles of the theory or whether they set the course that later leads to other, more immediate principles, it is these premises with which the question of reality convergence deals.

A reader can accept or reject the basic unsupported premises of a theory. The fact that a set of premises appears to be self-evident to a theorist does not mean that every reader will agree. Take, for example, Newman's expanding consciousness. If one holds a firm opinion that consciousness does not expand, then Newman's theory lacks reality convergence. Because the principle of expanding consciousness underlies the rest of the theory, none of it can be accepted if this basic principle is not accepted as a real statement about the human being.

Reality convergence has to do with whether or not the basic premises of a theory are accepted or rejected. Notice that this component of external criticism allows for more disagreement than is the case for most criteria of internal criticism. Although all readers would agree that the basic premises of a theory must be adequate to serve as a base for theory development (internal criticism), there is little likelihood that each reader will agree on whether or not any particular set of premises does or does not converge with reality.

Interpretation tells what sort of nursing world the theorist perceives. Does the theorist's perception conform with that of the reader? Johnson's world of behavior as the setting for nursing is a good example. Patient *behavior* simply does not reflect the world of nursing for many nurses.

Reality may refer to what is perceived to be man, health, or nursing. One critic might judge a theory to be deficient if it takes a reductionist view of *man*—for example, explaining him on the basis of stimuli and responses—if that critic has a conflicting, holistic view of man. Similarly, some critics may fault a theory for having an illness-based concept of *health* if they have a strong personal commitment to well care.

Judgments as to reality convergence also include disagreements about method. For example, some nurses will not accept a theory unless its conjoined method allows for empirical research by the so-called scientific method. These critics reject the dialectic methodology on this basis. Some would argue that it is possible to subject conclusions reached by dialectic reasoning to research in problematic or logistic modes. We will return to this notion in a later chapter.

In looking at the criterion of reality convergence, it is important to recognize that any given theory can be negated by viewing that theory in light of a different principle, interpretation, or method. If the critic *assumes* that a logistic approach is the only acceptable method, then she simply rejects every nonlogistic theory as failing to reflect reality. Similarly, a critic committed to a problematic method will reject a nonproblematic method. There is no higher court of appeals to which such basic disagreements can be referred.

Utility

The criterion of utility requires that a nursing theory be useful to the practitioner in her work, whether it be nursing practice, education, research, or administration. A nursing theory should structure the work, giving the practicing nurse a frame of reference from which to view patients and from which to make patient care decisions. For the nurse educator, a theory should provide the basis for curriculum organization as well as indicate appropriate methods of teaching. A theory has utility for the nurse researcher if it suggests important subject matter for investigation and appropriate methods of inquiry. It should guide the nurse administrator in the organization of the nursing department and delivery of nursing care services. If a theory is too esoteric to be applied in day-to-day operations and decisions, then it fails to meet the criterion of utility. People can disagree on what is useful, however. Newman's (1994) theory of health as expanding consciousness may seem totally inapplicable to many nurses, yet she gives a wealth of patient care examples that demonstrate how she finds it useful.

If a theory is to be usable, its selected concepts must take on meaning in the world of extant nursing activities. One might, for example, examine King's principle of transaction: an agreement reached between patient and nurse in relation to any subject matter. One might criticize this principle as lacking utility for the care of many patients (eg, the comatose, the irrational, or the newborn). Suppose King were to respond to this criticism with an argument that her theory was not meant to cover all nursing occasions. This would shift the argument from one of utility to one of scope.

Utility requires that the concepts of a theory be operationalized. Here some might take issue with Rogers's (1990, p. 8) principle of resonancy (continuous change from lower to higher frequency wave patterns in human and environmental fields). If a nurse could not conceptualize how that principle could direct her practice, it would lack utility. Another nurse might understand the principle in a way that allowed her to use it in clinical practice. The question of utility depends on who can use what and how.

To exhibit utility, a theory must direct work in extant settings. Its terms and concepts must be operationalized in ways that allow its application, and that application must facilitate the nursing activities rather than hinder them.

Significance

A theory meets the criterion of significance if it: (1) addresses essential, not peripheral, issues in nursing, and (2) contributes to the development of nursing knowledge. The first subcriterion of significance might be coined the *so what factor*. Often one hears a theory explained, finds no fault with its internal structure, sees its applicability to practice, yet is tempted to ask: So what? Usually this happens when the selected subject matter of the theory is peripheral to one's concept of what really matters in nursing. Because nursing is such a complex phenomenon, it is not surprising that some authors opt to deal with trivial concepts that are easily explained and manipulated. Nor is it surprising if people differ on what is or is not significant.

The second element contained in the criterion of significance is that of the theory's research potential, that is, its potential for expanding nursing knowledge. If a theory is significant, it lends itself to further nursing research. Ellis (1968) in a classic piece on characteristics of theories, notes:

> *Another characteristic of significant theories is that they are capable of generating a great deal of new information. Hypotheses which are highly probable may be so simply because they state what is apparent empirically and contribute little that is new. A theory that generates many hypotheses, even some without high probability, or some that are difficult to test, can contribute significantly to understanding. (p. 221)*

Sometimes, when theories are criticized as failing to lend themselves to research, the fault may lie in the critic's narrow view of research methods rather than in the theory itself. New perceptions on research methods have greatly enhanced the ability of many theories to undergo research.

The criterion of significance, then, is met when the research stemming from a theory has potential for predicting and controlling those factors that comprise the essential aspects of nursing. A significant theory addresses essential, not peripheral, phenomena.

Discrimination

Another important criterion for a nursing theory is its capacity to discriminate. Does the theory differentiate nursing from other health professions on the one hand and from other caring-tending acts on the other? A theory that discriminates bounds its subject matter definitively. Discrimination is important in a practice discipline that draws on knowledge from so many other fields. If, for example, the nurse is acting *as a nurse* and not as a pharmacologist when she administers a medication, the discriminating nursing theory will enable one to explain why. Similarly, one would be able to determine if a triage nurse were acting *as a nurse* or as a substitute physician.

No two theories include exactly the same phenomena within the given boundaries of nursing. The important point is that the boundaries be precise and clear, so that it is possible to make judgments, placing extant acts and practices inside or outside of the prescribed boundaries.

Two further criteria—scope and complexity—are important for external criticism of a theory although there is little consensus on them. Both may be seen as continuums, with various theorists opting for different placements on them.

Scope of Theory

Authors differ about whether a nursing theory should have a broad or limited scope (conceived of as two locations on the continuum). At one stage the argument tended to be either/or. Now most nurses recognize that there is place for theory development all along the continuum. The chief quality affected by scope is the depth of the theory. Simply put, a theory can be more detailed if it is designed to cover a limited practice—let's say gerontologic nursing—than when speaking for every kind of nursing imaginable.

The narrower the theory, the more potential it has for guidance; the broader the theory, the more global its terms and meanings, hence the less potential for guidance. The impossible ideal would be a theory that covered all kinds of nursing yet was highly detailed in its formulation. Today, there is much interest in mid-range theories because they are more easily researched than broader concepts.

The scope issue presses us to consider whether nursing is a single discipline or a combination of disciplines. Will nursing be able to develop a theory that functions optimally for such diverse nursing domains as public health, psychiatric nursing, and acute care nursing? Is it even necessary? The question of utility may interact with questions of scope. If a specific theory is more useful, should a nurse in a specialty practice be required to use a less effective wide-scope theory simply for conformity?

Complexity

The criterion of complexity opposes the criterion of parsimony. The argument *for* complexity in a theory is that it allows for explanation and interrelationship of more variables. Complexity enables a theory to account for the richness of its subject matter. The criterion of parsimony strives to limit theory elements, to streamline. Parsimony requires that the fewest possible variables be selected as descriptive and explanatory components. It has the advantage of clearly separating figure and background, of setting the critical elements of nursing in relief so that they are more easily perceived. Parsimony and complexity can be seen as opposite poles of a continuum.

At times a complex idea can be expressed in parsimonious terms. Einstein's basic theory ($E = Mc^2$) is parsimonious in the extreme, yet it represents a complex set of ideas. The balance between complexity and parsimony must be dictated by the inherent nature of the given theory.

OTHER EVALUATIVE CRITERIA

This book divides evaluative criteria into those appropriate for internal and external criticism. Other theory critics elaborate different lists of criteria and different methods for evaluating theories. The reader should explore these alternate formulations as well. Meleis (1997), for example, adds an interesting criterion called the circle of contagiousness (pp. 262–264). By this she means whether or not, and to what degree, a theory is adopted by others. This might be called the factor of geographic spread. Whether popularity and a theory's caliber coincide, only time will tell, but it is certainly a criterion worth assessing.

Chinn and Kramer (1983, pp. 128–139) have a parsimonious set of criteria for evaluating theories: clarity, simplicity, generality, accessibility, and importance. For these authors, clarity means essentially the same thing it means in this book. Their notion of simplicity refers to the number of components and relationships in a theory, and generality refers to the scope of events covered by the theory. Accessibility tests the extent to which empirical indicators can be identified and how attainable projected outcomes are. Importance refers to the extent to which the theory has clinical significance.

Fawcett (1993, pp. 39–45) uses the criteria of significance, internal consistency, parsimony, testability, empirical adequacy, and pragmatic adequacy. Whatever schema one elects to follow, the important thing is that a theory be seriously studied rather than accepted without deliberation.

SUMMARY

This chapter has examined the ways of passing judgment on a theory. One needs to differentiate between aspects of personal preference and elements of flawed thinking on the part of a theorist. Separating internal from external criticism assists in this endeavor. In addition, the separation encourages more rigorous thinking on the part of the evaluator. Criteria for both internal and external analysis exist. Performance on one criterion may affect other criteria. For example, if the clarity of a theory is poor, it may be impossible to evaluate other criteria with precision.

Personal preferences can bias one's evaluation of a theory. For example, a reader who detests the New Age movement may have difficulty suspending that judgment in reading a New Age theory. Not only can a reader have preferences concerning a theory, but she may have preferences concerning evaluative criteria. For example, different degrees of parsimony and complexity appeal to different people. None of this is to say that theories should not be judged. If nursing has erred, it has been in the failure to criticize. Criticism need not be seen in a negative light. A concise evaluation of the present formulation may be the first step in improving a theory.

REFERENCES

Chinn, P. L., & Kramer, M. K. (1991). *Theory and nursing: A systematic approach*. St. Louis: Mosby-Year Book.

Ellis, R. (1969, May/June). Characteristics of significant theories. *Nursing Research, 3*, 217–222.

Fawcett, J. (1993). *Analysis and evaluation of nursing theories*. Philadelphia: Davis.

Meleis, A. I. (1997). *Theoretical nursing: Development and progress* (3rd ed.). Philadelphia: Lippincott.

Newman, M. (1994). *Health as expanding consciousness* (2nd ed). New York: National League for Nursing Press.

Rubin, R. (1968, May/June). A theory of clinical nursing. *Nursing Research, 3*, 210–212.

Rogers, M. E. (1990). Nursing: Science of unitary, irreducible, human beings—Update 1990. In E. A. M. Barrett (Ed.), *Visions of Rogers' science-based nursing* (pp. 5–11). New York: National League for Nursing Press.

14 *Focus on Environment*

ENVIRONMENTAL ROOTS

Although every nursing theory, of necessity, reflects some notion of the patient's environment, in many environment is a key focus. Nurses often trace their interest in environment back to Florence Nightingale who was as much sanitary engineer (environmental engineer) as nurse. Much of the text in her *Notes on Nursing* (reissued 1992) is devoted to improvements in the patient's environment. For example, she speaks of the "health of houses," identifying five essential points: pure air, pure water, efficient drainage, cleanliness, and light (p. 14).

As Schuyler (1992) summarizes in that reissue:

> *Nightingale's concern for the health of others was not restricted to the Army. In the ten years after the Crimean War, she worked to reform civilian hospitals and workhouse infirmaries in England; to improve health and sanitation in India and other British colonies; and to establish the first professional schools for nurses and midwives. (p. 8)*

Environmental reform was the crux of most of these diverse activities. Although the meaning of *environment* changes with each nurse theorist, nurses have sustained that interest in environment ever since Nightingale. The environments that theorists address range from a community health perspective to a notion of mind as environment, from a perception of culture as the important environmental factor to a global concept of environment.

In this nation, public health nursing has always been associated with the environment. Early public health nurses dealt with environmental concerns not unlike those faced by Nightingale herself: unsanitary conditions, nutritional failures, industrial hazards, and ill health due to both poverty and ignorance.

Today we have two environmental models that follow in this tradition: the public health nursing model and the community health nursing model. Rothman (1990) differentiates between them this way:

> *Community health nursing practice concentrates on the direct care of individuals, families, and groups; the community is a client to the degree that it impacts on the direct care of individuals, families, and groups. Public health nursing is directed toward legal mandates to protect health and programs for specific segments of the population. . . .*
>
> *The public health nurse employs a method/process directed toward identification of high-risk groups and collaborates with multidisciplinary teams in planning and coordinating programs and services to address actual and potential health problems. (p. 418)*

Rothman differentiates nursing of people in communities from the nursing of substandard communities themselves. This to not say that everyone agrees with Rothman's differentiations. Nor do programs in public health always opt for one model to the exclusion of the other. In many educational programs—and community health programs as well—one finds combined models. Kuehnert (1995), for example, in his Interactive and Organizational Model of Community as Client tries to serve three masters:

> *The public health nursing agency targets three distinct community units in its practice, resulting in separate but interactive foci of practice for both staff and the agency. The community-wide focus of practice applies the nursing process to the community as a whole, so that public health nursing programs are directed to other units of the community, but the community as a whole is the overall target for health improvement or preservation. In the aggregate or group focus, both high-risk aggregates or subgroups of the community and organizations such as schools and workplaces are targeted. Individuals and their families, particularly those at risk for poor health outcomes or already experiencing health problems, are also a target of public health nursing. (p. 11)*

By whatever name, public health/community health nursing is one model of care that looks beyond the patient's immediate environment (the hospital, the home, the long-term care facility), that is, it sees environment as more than the place where he is physically housed. Three environmentally driven types of theory are discussed here: transcultural, multienvironmental, and feminist theory. These approaches share a conviction that a focus on a patient's immediate environment is not enough. All look beyond the sick room; beyond that agreement, they diverge radically.

TRANSCULTURAL NURSING

Leininger is credited with making transcultural nursing a major theme in nursing theory. With her anthropologic background, it is not surprising that she diagnosed nursing care to suffer when the nurse failed to appreciate the patient's culture and the meanings that culture attributes to illnesses and their treatment.

For Leininger, the cultural dimension is imposed on a strong commitment to a care philosophy. Welding the two concepts together, she made nurses aware of the importance of considering a patient's culture to help him. Leininger encouraged two trends in nursing: (1) a concentrated study of selected cultures by nurses intending to work with those populations, and (2) the development among nurses of a general sensitivity to the fact that all people have cultural patterns and meanings that should be considered in developing plans of care.

Many of Leininger's (1991) assumptive premises deal with the cultural aspect of nursing, including:

- *Every human culture has generic (lay, folk, or indigenous) care knowledge and practices and usually professional care knowledge and practices which vary transculturally.*
- *Clients who experience nursing care that fails to be reasonably congruent with the client's beliefs, values, and caring lifeways will show signs of cultural conflicts, noncompliance, stresses, and ethical or moral concerns. (p. 45)*

In her transcultural research, Leininger (1991) found:

- *There are more signs of diversities than universalities among the 54 cultures, and especially between Western and non-Western cultures.*
- *Culture care meanings and practices are difficult to tease out largely because they are embedded in the social structure, in non-Western cultures especially in kinship, religious beliefs, and political factors; whereas in Western cultures care is viewed largely as high-tech tasks, cost factors, political decisions, and problems with language to understand clients' care needs. (p. 57)*

Nurses educated in Leininger's and other transcultural programs have been sensitized to the needs of patients from other cultures. In a world that grows constantly smaller and more mobile, the message is timely. For these nurses, the patient's environment, namely, his culture, *is* the message, and if a nurse cannot read the message, care efforts may fail.

Leininger's (1991, p. 43) Sunrise model holds the nurse accountable for learning the patient's world view, including: technological factors, religious and philosophical factors, kinship and social factors, cultural values and lifeways, political and legal factors, economic factors, and educational factors. The vulnerability in this theory is that this may be asking the impossible for a nurse from a metropolitan area who may see people from numerous and diverse ethnic communities in a single day, under the press of delivering rapid care.

Leininger may be seen as giving more credence to the environmental background than to individual characteristics that may or may not conform to the patient's background. Unlike many feminist theorists, Leininger accepts the patient's environment as a given, not as a domain for intensive intervention and change.

THE TOTAL HUMAN ENVIRONMENT

Levine (1989) provides a more intimate, body-based view of a human's environment, consisting of (1) the living tissue environment (eg, microorganisms, pollutants, and other unperceived impacting phenomena), (2) the sensory environment (eg, energies of things such as light, sound, touch), and (3) the conceptual environment (aspects of being such as thought, ideas, and language). Part of her notion of environment is internal, part external. There is an historical element as well. Levine says that:

> . . . active participation by the individual requires a genetic endowment specific to a specific habitat. Thus the fundamental nature of adaptation is a consequence of a historical progression: the evolution of the species through time, reflecting the sequence of change in the genetic patterns that have recorded the change in the historical environments. That history is recorded in living cells and living systems of cells, a history so various that only the most obvious events can be identified. (p. 327)

In comparing Levine and Leininger, one sees how diverse the conceptions of environment may be. Yet, however it is cast, environment has always been one of the major commonplaces to be considered in evaluating a nursing theory. Feminists move us to yet another perception of environment.

FEMINIST THEORY IN NURSING

Ashley (1977) is credited as having had a major role in bringing feminist issues to the attention of nurses. Her feminism is based on seeing the physician and hospital administrator (cast as men in her writing) as keeping nursing repressed through a mode of paternalism.

Ashley paints her villains dark. As she maintained concerning physicians in her classic work on the subject:

> *Despite the sometimes antisocial tactics used by physicians to maintain their control, sociologists and the public have idealized them, helping them maintain their public image as the perfect professionals.*
>
> *Although organized medicine has both created and perpetuated social problems of major significance, the public is still encouraged to accept medical paternalism and to look up to doctors as final authorities on matters of health and illness. (p. 124)*

Although this raillery sounds old-fashioned today, it was a unique view of the hospital as environment—and an antifeminist environment—in Ashley's day. After Ashley, nursing was never without its feminist concerns. Yet the notion of environment soon spread from a view of the hospital to a view of the society and then the world.

One would imagine that a profession so heavily dominated by women would be ripe for feminist concerns, yet the connections between nursing and feminist organizations have often been testy. The nonnursing feminist press and major feminist organizations have often condemned nursing for its conservatism, or worse, suggested that ambitious women would select medicine over nursing as a career goal.

Some feminists perceive an inherent conflict between the values of feminism and the values expressed in caring. Condon (1992, p. 17) explains the feminist concern that any feminine role perceived as following a caring model puts the carers at risk of exploitation by those for whom they care, thereby reinforcing the oppressive expectation that women should be selfless carers.

Nevertheless, the voice of feminism is alive and well in nursing, with its members voicing positions ranging from modest to radical. Moccia (1990) advocates a strong feminist base for nursing, challenging the profession in this manner:

> *If nurses are to become active participants in bringing society to a new reality, if we are to fulfill the role of transformative intellectuals, then we will have to redefine ourselves and our institutions. As we find ways to break the tentacles of the patriarchy and to erode its base, we will obviously find ourselves in new relationships. (p. 75)*

Often the feminist position has a sense of rage underlying its positions and theories. Moccia (1990) illustrates this point:

> *There is too much that is unconscionable and cries out for relief—so much that we are left shaking and trembling and close to being paralyzed by moral outrage. The dark motif of the patriarchy encourages a sense*

of futility, desperation, and of irreparable ruptures between private lives
and public actions. (p. 76)

Feminist philosophies espouse the importance of gender equity
and try to raise the social consciousness of women and men in recognizing sexist inequities in the society. The inequities addressed are
as variable as are the countries in which feminists speak, write, and
become politically active.

The use of sexist language has been one of the tamer themes,
and Sampsell (1990) discusses the subject in typical feminist fashion:

> *The patriarchal view of woman as a subspecies of man shows readily*
> *in the contemporary experience. Common language is rife with examples*
> *such as the generic use of man and masculine pronouns to represent*
> *all human beings (eg, the paradigm that depicts nursing expertise in*
> *the areas of Man, Health and Environment); the lack of gender fairness*
> *(eg, man and woman are parallel terms, whereas man and wife defines*
> *the man as an individual and the woman only in relationship to him)*
> *and the negative connotation reserved for words that depict feminine*
> *traits. . . . (p. 244)*

Creating a sensitivity to language is on most feminist agendas,
but political action to right societal insults against women is a
higher priority.

Ecofeminism

One version of feminism combines the feminist perspective with an
ecological viewpoint (ecofeminism). From an ecofeminist perspective, what is cared for, cared about, is the planet, the earth itself,
including its populations. The proposed solutions advocate advancing feminist power and preserving ecology at the same time. Obviously, the ecological and the feminist viewpoints can be separated
and in many cases are. However, we see a strong tendency to combine
the two factions.

In most versions, the ecofeminist viewpoint is not set in the so-
called New Age world paradigm; instead its ideology represents a
counterculture position against the social, political factions in power
in various governments worldwide. Although the position is coined
against the acts of these ruling powers, the view of the world (context
in our terms) is similar. Those in power and the feminists see the same
world; they simply would like it to be managed in different ways.

Kleffel (1991, p. 7) describes the ecofeminist position as one
that sees the fate of the human species and the planet at stake. She
postulates that no male-led revolution will counteract the present
horrors of overpopulation and destruction of natural resources. This

linked concern for the natural world and for the abuses of a male-run society is typical of the ecofeminist position.

Some nurses are uncomfortable with the tactics of assertive feminists. True, some feminists can be strident, taking positions that seem harsh. These feminists would claim that their tactics are shaped by today's world and that they have little choice if they are to make an impact. Feminist choices involve not only matters of tactics but selections of themes as well. As has ever been the case, it is not always possible to serve a larger cause and the individual simultaneously. Where a choice must be made, many nurses in the feminist camp opt for the macrocosmic view over the one-to-one-ideology.

Many nurse ecofeminists (or simply feminists) decry the fact that the typical nursing theory takes a one nurse-to-one patient perspective. They object to environment being conceived merely as the patient's immediate surroundings. These positions, they assert, narrow one's perspective and keep nursing from addressing its true subject matter: the larger social, political, and ecological, global picture. This feminist perspective makes political reform the immediate, not a tangential aim of nursing, and this represents a radical change in content, context, and goals from other theories we have examined.

Feminists: Not All Alike

Kleffel (1991, p. 7) differentiates four types of contemporary feminism—liberal feminism, radical feminism, traditional Marxist feminism, and socialist feminism. Her list should remind us that feminists, even among nurses, are not all of a kind. It is true, however, that some of the feminists once classified as Marxist or socialist have shifted their interest to the ecological, not surprising in a world where so many communist and socialist states have fallen, bringing the political form into question.

The linking of a feminist agenda to an ecological agenda simply broadens feminist goals. The earlier focus on gender equity has not been sacrificed. Indeed, the growing sensitivity to harassment in the workplace has increased the zeal of this pursuit by most feminists. Battling violence against women worldwide remains a major effort on the feminist plate. Another issue of major importance—the lack of attention given to women's diseases or women's fate when contracting diseases—has received an important boost by requirements that federally sponsored research include women as study subjects.

Whatever the focus, ecology, women's rights, women's health, societal failures, many feminists of all persuasions focus on political action. They recognize that government is the major decision-maker on these issues. For many feminist nurses, the appropriate subject matter (content) for nursing is politics. Achieving the desired political world is seen as prior to and prerequisite for the hands-on care that is the first concern in most nursing theories.

Not all feminists perceive the political as the only or proper domain for intervention. Henderson (1997) stresses that the central theme should be consciousness raising for women.

Trippet and Bryson (1995) join consciousness raising and women's health together in a model of health care that focuses on both positive and negative domains of roles, image, sensory deprivation, mobility, hormonal influences and sexuality, nutrition, economic issues, abuse, and depression. Certainly, the feminist movement has been central in making women's health a specialty and advancing its growth.

The expansion of the women's health movement is a positive feature associated with feminism, but criticism has been leveled against the movement as well. The failure of feminists to focus first and foremost on the quality of one-to-one care is confusing to some nurses who have internalized that role as their chief function. Although most nurses support feminist goals, many would assert that feminist politics, worthy though they may be, simply are not nursing. Other nurses are bothered by the fact that some feminist groups favor political revolution to reform, but feminist groups are far from agreement on their political goals and tactics.

Many people think of feminist theories as holistic, but that is not always the case. The confusion is probably because their common subject matter (the state of the country or world) seems large. But their approach is seldom holistic. Instead, feminists seem interested in analyzing the parts (political decisions), analyzing the infrastructures of a society, and intervening in them—a view in which the whole is known through its parts.

In contrast, Marxist feminists, where they are consistent to original Marxian principles, may follow a dialectic thought pattern in which the world is seen as evolving, moving through an inevitable series of thesis, antithesis, and synthesis. Moccia is a good example of a feminist who is sensitive to the dialectic thought process. Many others, however, have assumed the feminist causes without adopting the Hegelian/Marxist dialectic.

Postmodernism and Feminism

Some authors criticize nurse feminists for being simplistic and casting all women in the same role, with the same labels. As Miller (1997) says:

Postmodern feminists acknowledge that because women's experiences vary along so many axes (age, race-ethnicity, class, sexual identification, and so on), it is impossible to describe those experiences under one theory without ignoring the significant differences among women. Just as women are not one but many, so feminisms and feminist theories must be plural, partial, multiple, contingent, local and small scale. Feminists postmodernists also try to avoid the privileging of one axis over another, seeking instead complex multiple locations and identities of women's lives. They acknowledge diversity among women and the possibility of the coexistence of many feminisms. (p. 149)

The postmodern perspective argues against universal feminist themes, favoring local, contextual efforts tailored to each specific situation and group of women.

SUMMARY

Many nursing theories concentrate on environment, starting with Nightingale, leading forward into our own times. Environment, which we have sometimes called context in this book, is related to the patient's internal and external environments; the political, social, and gender roles; and ecological environments.

Many environmental theories (from Nightingale to the feminists) could be characterized as crusader theories. They aim to change things, whatever the environment that is pursued. Other theories (like transcultural nursing) are more passive—accepting and generally working within the patient's given environment.

The present era is ripe for the development of environmental theories of nursing, particularly in an era when care is being distributed over many settings other than the acute care hospital. Today's student and today's nurse may find themselves delivering care in environments that have been not been addressed for decades (if ever), and they may need to consider more kinds and aspects of environment than occurred in previous care-delivery models.

REFERENCES

Ashley, J. A. (1977). *Hospitals, paternalism, and the role of the nurse.* New York: Teachers College Press.

Condon, E. H. (1992, January/February). Nursing and the caring metaphor: Gender and political influences on an ethics of care. *Nursing Outlook, 1,* 14–19.

Henderson, D. J. (1997). Conscious-raising as a feminist nursing action: Promise and practice, present, and future. In S. E. Thorne & V. E. Hayes (Eds.), *Nursing praxis: Knowledge and action* (pp. 157–179). Thousand Oaks, CA: Sage.

Kleffel, D. (1991). An ecofeminist analysis of nursing knowledge. *Nursing Forum, 4,* 5–18.

Kuehnert, P. L. (1995, February). The interactive and organizational model of community as client: A model for public health nursing practice. *Public Health Nursing, 1,* 9–17.

Leininger, M. M. (1991). The theory of culture care diversity and universality. In M. M. Leininger (Ed.), *Culture care diversity & universality: A theory of nursing* (pp. 5–68). New York: National League for Nursing Press.

Levine, M. E. (1980). The conservation principles of nursing: Twenty years later. In J. Riehl-Sisca (Ed.), *Conceptual models for nursing practice* (3rd ed., pp. 325–337). New York: Appleton-Century-Crofts.

Miller, S. (1997). Multiple paradigms for nursing: Postmodern feminisms. In S. E. Thorne & V. E. Hayes (Eds.), *Nursing praxis: Knowledge and action* (pp. 140–156). Thousand Oaks, CA: Sage.

Moccia, P. (1990, March/April). Re-claiming our communities. *Nursing Outlook, 2,* 73–76.

Nightingale, F. (1992). *Notes on nursing* (reissue). Philadelphia: Lippincott.

Rothman, N. L. (1990, November). Toward description: Public health nursing and community health nursing are different. *Nursing & Health Care, 9,* 481–483.

Sampsell, C. M. (1990, Winter). The influence of feminist philosophy on nursing practice. *Image, 4,* 243–247.

Schuyler, C. B. (1992). Florence Nightingale. In F. Nightingale, with D. P. Carroll (Ed.), *Notes on nursing* (reissue), Philadelphia: Lippincott.

Trippet, S. E., & Bryson, M. R. (1995). A model of women's health nursing. *Health Care for Women International, 16,* 31–41.

15 *Common Themes in Nursing Theory*

This chapter summarizes and examines the common themes in grand nursing theory—not in an attempt to synthesize them, but to identify the different subject matters and approaches. We produce a map of topics and viewpoints, not a theory of nursing. The questions to be asked are: What can be gained by taking this subject matter or this approach for nursing theory? Which topics and which approaches are compatible and which contradictory if used within a single theory formulation?

SUBJECT MATTER OF NURSING THEORY

Most theories take as their primary subject matter the human being (the patient), the nurse, environment, health, or their interfaces. Variations on these themes include the nursing act, the human–environment relationship, man in groups, the person in organizations, the human as he participates in God, and the health care system—to name a few. Each of these subject matters can be perceived in an infinite number of ways.

Human Being-Centered Theories of Nursing

An underlying assumption in human being-centered theories of nursing is that to know the human is to be able to infer what nursing is required. A major question for theories with this theme is whether nursing's subject matter is the *total* man or some *component* of his being. Furthermore, if nursing is applied to the total human, one must ask if that means man as an indivisible whole or if it means all the units comprising his totality (eg, psyche and soma; psychological, physiologic, and spiritual components; the various body systems taken together; the human's structure and function; or some other variation on his components). If, however, nursing is responsible for only some (but not all) components, which components fall inside of nursing's domain?

Human-centered theories also should declare *when* the total or partial human requires nursing. In some theories a person is labeled a patient when a health deficiency occurs. Other theories expand the category to include persons vulnerable to health deficits not yet manifest. Some theories consider every living person as patient for a lifetime. In many New Age theories, for example, nursing is an act of assisting in human development (expanding consciousness, extending self-mastery). These theories imply that nursing is an ongoing activity that one needs at every phase of life, regardless of the particular health status. When nursing is seen as always applicable, it tends to be equated with meeting all human needs. In other cases it is tightly tied to developmental needs, with "needs" being interpreted from traditional patterns like Erikson (1963) to transpersonal patterns like Wilber (1980, 1986). Boundary issues arise here if nurses fail to differentiate themselves from others who also might see themselves as guardians of development—psychiatrists, developmental psychologists, transpersonal psychologists, or clergymen for a start.

When the need for nursing is perceived as intermittent, it is usually limited to the meeting of health-related needs. A theory should identify the phenomena that initiate the need for nursing (eg, stress or strain, disequilibrium or ineffective adaptation, a deficit, incapacity, dysfunctional or deviant behavior, disharmony, disease, etc).

Sometimes it is not the individual who is the subject matter of a theory. There are numerous *plural man* theories in which a theorist claims that her patient is a group or community. When only one of these alternatives is singled out, the theorist is usually on firm ground. But when the person, people in groups, *and* humans in larger society are all asserted to be legitimate subjects of the same theory, the claim is seldom delivered on. Often this slogan, once said, is ignored. Suppose, for example, that a theorist's patient is defined by his disequilibrium. Does she ever tell how to recognize disequilibrium in a group or community? Are her examples of care applicable to the larger sense of patient or only to the one-on-one situation? It is not wrong to have a subject matter of plural man, but it *is* wrong if it is not carried out in the resultant theory.

Human–Other Units as Theory Subject Matter

In human–other units, man is still the subject matter, but he is seen through his blending with and participation in something else. The "other" with which the human is combined may be any sort of social, political, geographic, or conceptual entity. Man in relation to family is one such unit. Man as a family member (husband, father, mother, child) would comprise one such human–other unit. In other cases, the entire family unit becomes the patient (rather than any member of it singled out). The psychiatric nurse therapist, for example, might take the family as a whole as her unit of analysis and therapy. For a comparative view of different approaches to family therapy, see Whall (1980). The same difference applies to notions of public health/ community health nursing. The person in the community is a man–other unit, whereas the community as patient could qualify as an environmental theory instead. Sometimes the conjoined unit is much larger than the man–family or person–community unit. Human–environment or even man–universe theories are popular. The new paradigm theories specialize in these "larger than life" perspectives. Newman's (1994) theory of man participating in a larger evolving consciousness is one example. Some religious theories take a similar perspective; Longway's (1970) focus on the human–God interface could qualify here. In man–other theories, nursing may prescribe intervention in either man, the "other," or both.

The Nurse as Subject Matter

Some theories take the nurse rather than the patient as the focal subject matter. The approach varies widely, from looking at roles performed, to identifying tasks, to examining the nurse's motivation. It is not uncommon for theorists who use an operational methodology to view nursing in terms of role, and it is not uncommon for caring theories to view the nurse through her motivation. The nursing process identifies the nurse through what she does, that is, her activities, both intellectual and psychomotor. When nonnurses study nursing, they frequently equate nursing with the psychomotor tasks that are self-evident and open to observation.

Sometimes the nurse is defined by her credentials or licenses—as a registered professional nurse, as a baccalaureate prepared nurse, as certified midwife, for example. This is a legalistic answer to the problem of definition. Other times, *nurse* is perceived to include all members of the nursing staff (aides, practical nurses). In some theories the term *nurse* may be applied to anyone who completes acts of a specified nature, with or without educational or experiential qualifications.

Considering Patient and Nurse Together

It is common, though not essential, that the patient and the nurse act out of reciprocal, complementary principles. For example, Johnson's (1980) patient is motivated by a disturbance in one or more behavioral systems, perhaps a frustrated drive. Her nurse, reciprocally, is an external regulatory force who aims to restore or attain behavioral system balance and stability by manipulating the patient's drives and needs.

In Levine's (1989) theory, the patient *adapts* while the nurse *conserves* (she conserves those patient adaptations that are seen as productive). In Hall's (1966) theory, the nurse *mirrors* (reflects back the patient's own feelings), the patient *masters* (his feelings, his self-control).

In Roy's (1989) theory, the patient *responds to stimuli*, whereas the nurse *manipulates stimuli*. Even Orlando's (1990) theory has reciprocal principles, if a bit more complicated than many of the theories discussed above. The nurse observes the patient's behavior, interprets it, then checks her reaction with the patient. Only after the patient confirms or clarifies the meaning of the behavior does she act on the behavior to solve the patient's problem. We could shorten the system as: patient action, nurse reaction, nurse–patient validation, and nurse action.

In a few theories, the patient and the nurse operate on the same principle rather than complementary principles. In Orem's (1985) theory, for example, both act out of self-care agency. The nurse's justification for taking over the patient's self-care is the patient's incapacity to do so. The principle from which they act, however, remains the same: self-care.

A few theories focus so exclusively on one polarity of the relationship (either the patient or the nurse) that they say little about the other aspect. For example, Rogers's work focuses primarily on the patient, that is, the nature of what it is to be a human being (unitary man). Rogers's (1990) principles (resonancy, helicy, integrality) rest in unitary man, not in the nurse as nurse nor in the nursing act (as discrete from other human actions).

In contrast, Benner's (1984, pp. 44–46) theory focuses on the nurse, not the patient, identifying the following domains of nursing practice: (1) the helping role, (2) the teaching-coaching function, (3) the diagnostic and patient-monitoring function, (4) managing effectively the rapidly changing situations, (5) administering and monitoring therapeutic interventions and regimens, (6) monitoring and ensuring the quality of health care practices, and (7) maintaining organizational and work-role competencies. Although these actions rest in the nurse, they are not principles as was the case in the examples cited earlier. Benner, Tanner, and Chesla (1996) elaborate on Benner's theory.

For most theories, it is possible to represent the nurse–patient relationship as a sequential triad: (1) the patient's undesirable, initial status, (2) the nursing act, and (3) the patient's desirable status (goal or end point). Some examples follow:

Hall
1. Decreased self-control
2. Mirroring-nurturing
3. Self-mastery

Levine
1. Disequilibrium
2. Conservation
3. Equilibrium

Roy
1. Responses exceeding the adaptation level
2. Manipulation of stimuli
3. Responses within the adaptation level

Orem
1. (Decreased) self-care
2. (Substituted) self-care
3. (Resumed) self-care

These triads shift from patient to nurse to patient. When the patient also assists in effecting his cure or care, such as with Levine's patient, one could build another triad exclusive to the patient. For Levine's patient, that would be: (1) disequilibrium, (2) adaptation, and (3) equilibrium.

In the New Paradigm

The new paradigm theories often do not show such a shift in principle from patient to nurse; the patient retains control. Instead, as Watson (1988) says, "The agent of change in this work is viewed as the individual patient, but the nurse can be a coparticipant in change through the human care process" (p. 74). Or as Quinn (1992, pp. 28, 34) claims, the nurse is the midwife to healing; she is an environment for the patient, a space where there the resonance of two people interacts during healing. Theories in the new paradigm see the patient as the main agent, the nurse as helper. Some few New Age theories would be classified as patient focused, but the newer ones usually focus on the interaction (like Quinn and Watson). Even with a focus on the interaction, the patient is weightier than the nurse. The nurse helps build the interaction, but the patient remains captain of the relationship. Quinn's midwife example describes the power relations of the situation.

Every nursing theory has a focus. Is the author interested in telling nurses what to do? Or in understanding the patient? These are not incompatible goals, but typically one aspect is stressed over the other. Where the patient is the focus, the theorist implies that adequate knowledge of the patient makes the necessary nursing care self-evident. In a physiologically based conceptualization of the patient, this thesis is evident. On the whole, patient-based theories have a humanitarian appeal because they begin and end with the patient.

Theories that rest heavily on the nursing side of the equation often have actional principles. They have intrinsic appeal for the young nurse learner because they give strong directives, that is, they tell her what to do. Most theories of this sort deal with the nurse's overt actions; others focus instead on her thought processes.

Theories in the new paradigm show an interesting development in relation to the patient–nurse duality. Originally, most focused heavily on the nature of man, like Rogers's (1970) original work. Now the theories have developed in two directions, some focusing on the nature of the interrelationship between patient and nurse (Parse, 1981; Watson, 1988), others developing sets of nursing interventions (Dossey, 1997; Dossey, Keegan, Guzzetta, & Kolkmeier, 1995; Quinn, 1988, 1996). In what appears to be a more rapid pace, these latter theories are following the same sequence of development as the nursing process/diagnosis/intervention theory.

Nurse–Patient Interaction as Subject Matter

One important aspect of the nurse–patient linkage deals with interpretation. Although it is legitimate for the nurse to act on different principles than does the patient, it is not legitimate for her to be a creature from a different planet. Take for example a case in which the patient is explained entirely in terms of determinism (all his acts are results of what happened previously) yet the nurse is seen as operating out of a free will (not based on prior antecedents).

The critical questions are: Who is the nurse? What is the nursing act? Who or what is the patient? In what way do the two interface? Which of them, if either, is the dominant theme in the given theory?

Interaction theories take as their subject matter the conceptual product of the patient–nurse exchange. In King's (1981) theory, the ultimate principle of *transaction* arises between patient and nurse in the midst of their agreements. In Watson's (1988) theory, a transcendent coming together is possible. In both of these illustrations, the principle attaches to the interaction, not to the patient or the nurse.

Leininger's (1991, pp. 41–42) theory is an interesting variation on the interaction theme. Like Roy's theory, Leininger's rests heavily on the nurse's autonomous decision-making (she preserves/maintains, accommodates/negotiates, repatterns/restructures). Yet there is a requisite interaction of an unusual sort. It is not between nurse and patient, but between two competing health care systems: the care of the folkways and the care of the professional caregivers. For Leininger's system to work, the professionals must resolve differences between their system and the lay system—sort of a negotiation, with the professionals negotiating from strength (their knowledge of both systems).

Environment as Subject Matter

At times, environment is taken as the primary subject matter of nursing theory. How the environment is seen can be radically different from one theory to another. It could be a community, a given social class, a health care system, a political system, or the whole earth.

In some community health approaches, a neighborhood becomes the patient, that is, the direct recipient of the nursing actions. The political structure might be the subject matter of a feminist theory or even the planet in ecofeminism.

Most nursing theories consider environment as background rather than primary subject matter. Yet some feminist theory and public health conceptualizations place the environment front and center. In both of these cases, the larger unit rather than the hands-on care comprise the crux of the matter. It is assumed that resolving the macrolevel problems (however envisioned) will deter the ongoing need for one-to-one care. Nursing administration theories may take the health care organization as primary subject matter although such theories are hardly meant to replace caregiving models.

Health as Theory Subject Matter

It is rare for *health* itself to be the primary subject of a nursing theory; usually it is a goal. A comprehensive theory of health may include all aspects of health on a continuum from illness to wellness. Some theories focus only on the ill-health end of that continuum. These, like Orem's theory, justify the need for a nurse by a patient's deficit.

One common tactic is to view health as some sort of equilibrium (eg, homeostasis or homeokinesis). In models of this sort, adaptation (whatever is done to restore equilibrium) may be perceived as the function of the patient, the nurse, or both. What is kept in equilibrium may vary from physiologic to psychological to sociologic to spiritual. Johnson's theory is an equilibrium model in which the subject matter (behavioral equilibrium) is unique.

One form of the equilibrium–disequilibrium theory is the theory that takes stress as its major theme. Usually theories of this sort differentiate the stressor (source) from the strain (the result in the patient). Scott, Oberst, and Dropkin (1980) interpret stress in a cognitively based theory:

> . . . the individual's interpretation and evaluation of a stimulus-filled environment becomes the basis for a response to the stress experience, and in which emotions and physiological responses are viewed as by-products of cognition. (p. 11)

Chrisman and Riehl-Sisca (1989) have a more traditional definition of stress:

> It is important to distinguish the components of the stress process. The term stressor is useful to identify the agent that provokes the stress state. It is not a case, although it may be a catalyst or a crucial aspect of the cause. The stress or force that produces the stress state may originate from the stressor or from the organism (patient) itself. (p. 281)

Newer paradigms are more likely to see health as a state of continuous human evolution to higher levels, however defined. Fitzpatrick (1983) and Newman (1994) are more goal driven than some (toward faster rhythms or more expanded consciousness, respectively). Even Watson (1988), who progresses at a less frenetic pace, says that "The person has one basic striving: to actualize the real self, thereby developing the spiritual essence of the self, and in the highest sense, to become more Godlike" (p. 57).

In today's changing health care environment, discussions of types of health care are emerging as health care becomes distributed among diverse care organizations. For example, one sees more focus on topics of convalescent care, subacute care, or ambulatory care versus acute care. As these themes emerge, we can expect to see new theories of health directed along these lines of discrimination.

Recapping on Subject Matter

One way to look at themes in nursing theory is to examine the subject matters selected by theorists. We have identified six subject matters: (1) the human being (as patient), (2) man as a component of some larger, more encompassing unit, (3) the nurse or nursing act, (4) nurse–patient interactions, (5) environment, and (6) health. Although not all inclusive, these subject matters (the patient, the nurse, the environment, and health) dominate in the majority of nursing theories. One hears the common claim that all nursing theories are alike because they address these same subject matters, but the claim is deceiving.

APPROACHES TO THE NURSING DOMAIN

In addition to looking at what constitutes the nursing subject matter, it is important to characterize the theorist's perception of that domain. Although many classification schemes are possible, it is useful to sort nursing theories according to the character of the nursing act in relation to the patient. This classification allows for the following organization of nursing theories: (1) intervention, (2) conservation, (3) substitution, (4) sustenance/support, and (5) enhancement.

In an *intervention theory*, the nurse actively selects variables (in the patient or in the environment) for manipulation to bring about a determined change in the present state. The change to be desired is determined by the nurse, typically using her knowledge of health, societal norms, or both. Roy (1989) and Johnson (1988) exemplify this approach.

In intervention theories, action and decision-making rest heavily on the nurse as a professional. The patient is treated as the object of nursing rather than as a participant in the determination of his care. References to patient participation, when they occur, tend to be slogans rather than intrinsic to theory development. Ultimately, the nurse determines and executes the proper manipulation to bring about the desired change. Intervention theories rely on the concept of professional expertise exercised by the nurse.

A *conservation theory* aims to preserve those beneficial aspects of the patient's present situation, especially those beneficial aspects threatened by illness, problems, or (in the case of preventive care) potential problems. Levine's (1989) model is a good example of a conservation theory. Some public health theories rest on a conservation theory. In an era of growing public awareness of a person's responsibility for his own health, a conservation theory may provide a good fit with the social environment.

In contrast to the conservation theory, a *substitution theory* does not aim to preserve what exists, but to substitute for those capabilities the patient is no longer able to execute. Here agency resides with the patient, and nursing is a substitute for the patient's own will/intent. Agency moves from patient to nurse during the patient's incapacity.

Most substitution theories stress that the substitution be controlled, that the patient exercise his will and physical control to the greatest possible or logical extent. Undesired substitution is not inflicted on him. Nursing supplied in the absence of communication of patient intent is perceived as being what the patient would desire were he able to communicate that desire. In most substitution theories, the nurse is the patient's agent; she does not superimpose her own values, goals, and judgments for his when he is able to express them. Orem (1985) is a good example of an author who advocates a substitution theory.

Intervention and substitution theories reveal the polarities of the nurse–patient agency question, with intervention resting on the nursing agency of the professional, substitution resting on patient agency. The conservation theory bridges this polarity: agency rests with the nurse, but she conserves what already is inherent in the patient.

The *sustenance/support theory* is less concerned with affecting the course of an illness per se. Instead, it focuses on enabling the patient to better endure the passage of the health insult. Focus is on building coping mechanisms (both psychological and physiologic) and strengthening the ego function. Rubin (1968) exemplifies a sustenance theory. She sees the goal of nursing as ego maintenance in a stressful dependency situation (p. 210). The nursing care required is determined by the degree to which the patient can or cannot cope (unassisted) with a situation at any given point.

An *enhancement theory* of nursing is one that sees nursing as a means of improving the quality of the patient's existence, either in total, in relation to health, or in relation to some specified aspect of his being. Hall (1966), Rogers (1970, 1990), Watson (1988), and Newman (1994) exemplify enhancement theories. Most enhancement theories are dialectic, developmental, existential, or some combination of these elements. Enhancement theories share the perception that nursing enables the patient to emerge from the health insult (in some way) stronger, better, or improved because of having experienced or overcome the health insult.

Like an intervention theory, an enhancement theory aims to produce a change for the better. Unlike the intervention theory, the nature of that enhancement remains internal to the patient rather than being specifically determined and characterized in advance by the nurse.

SUMMARY

This chapter has reviewed common topics of and approaches to nursing theory. Even the limited commonplaces discussed here indicate the width of perspectives and diversity of topics one finds in nursing. Taken together, these topics represent the dominant approaches to the study of grand nursing theory today. The areas most likely to expand are the New Age theories and environment as subject matter.

REFERENCES

Benner, P. (1984). *From novice to expert: Excellence and power in clinical nursing practice.* Menlo Park, CA: Addison-Wesley.

Benner, P., Tanner, C. A., & Chesla, C. A. (1996). *Expertise in nursing practice: Caring, clinical judgment, and ethics.* New York: Springer.

Chrisman, M. K., & Riehl-Sisca, J. (1989). The systems-developmental-stress model. In J. Riehl-Sisca (Ed.), *Conceptual models for nursing practice* (3rd ed., pp. 277–295). Norwalk, CT: Appleton & Lange.

Dossey, B. M. (Ed.). (1997). *Core curriculum for holistic nursing.* Gaithersburg, MD: Aspen.

Dossey, B. M., Keegan, L., Guzzetta, C. E., & Kolkmeier, L. G. (Eds.). (1995). *Holistic nursing: A handbook for practice* (2nd ed.), Gaithersburg, MD: Aspen.

Erikson, E. H. (1963). *Childhood and society* (2nd ed., reissued with 1985 afterthought). New York: Norton.

Fitzpatrick, J. (1983). A life perspective rhythm model. In J. Fitzpatrick & A. Whall (Eds.), *Conceptual models of nursing: Analysis and application* (pp. 295–302). Bowie, MD: Robert J. Brady.

Hall, L. E. (1966). Another view of nursing care and quality. In K. M. Straub & K. S. Parker (Eds.), *Continuity of patient care: The role of nursing* (pp. 47–66). Washington, DC: Catholic University Press.

Johnson, D. E. (1980). The behavioral system model for nursing. In J. P. Riehl & C. Roy (Eds.), *Conceptual models for nursing practice* (2nd ed., pp. 207–216). New York: Appleton-Century-Crofts.

King, I. (1981). *A theory for nursing: Systems, concepts, process.* New York: Wiley.

Leininger, M. M. (1991). The theory of culture care diversity and universality. In M. M. Leininger (Ed.), *Culture care: Diversity & universality: A theory of nursing* (pp. 5–68). New York: National League for Nursing Press.

Levine, M. E. (1989). The conservation principles of nursing: Twenty years later. In J. Riehl-Sisca (Ed.), *Conceptual models for nursing practice* (3rd ed., pp. 325–337). New York: Appleton-Century-Crofts.

Longway, I. (1970, February/March). Toward a philosophy of nursing. *Journal of Adventist Education, 3,* 20–27.

Newman, M. (1994). *Health as expanding consciousness.* New York: National League for Nursing Press.

Orem, D. E. (1985). *Nursing concepts of practice* (3rd. ed.). New York: McGraw-Hill.

Orlando, I. J. (1990). *The dynamic nurse-patient relationship.* New York: National League for Nursing Press.

Parse, R. R. (1981). *Man-living-health: A theory of nursing.* New York: Wiley.

Quinn, J. (1988). Building a body of knowledge: Research on therapeutic touch. *Journal of Holistic Nursing, 1,* 37–45.

Quinn, J. (1996). *Therapeutic touch: A home study course for family caregivers: Everyone a healer.* [Videotape]. New York: National League for Nursing Press.

Quinn, J. F. (1992, July). Holding sacred space: The nurse as healing environment. *Holistic Nursing Practice, 4,* 26–36.

Rogers, M. E. (1970). *An introduction to the theoretical basis of nursing.* Philadelphia: Davis.

Rogers, M. E. (1990). Nursing: Science of unitary, irreducible, human beings—Update 1990. In E. A. M. Barrett (Ed.), *Visions of Rogers's science-based nursing* (pp. 1–11). New York: National League for Nursing Press.

Roy, C. (1989). The Roy adaptation model. In J. Riehl-Sisca (Ed.), *Conceptual models for nursing practice* (3rd ed., pp. 105–114). Norwalk, CT: Appleton & Lange.

Rubin, R. (1968, May/June). A theory of clinical nursing. *Nursing Research, 3,* 210–212.

Scott, D. W., Oberst, M. T., & Dropkin, M. J. (1980, October). A stress-coping model. *Advances in Nursing Science, 1,* 9–24.

Watson, J. (1988). *Nursing: Human science and human care.* New York: National League for Nursing Press.

Whall, A. L. (1980, October). Congruence between existing theories of family functioning and nursing theories. *Advances in Nursing Science, 1,* 59–68.

Wilber, K. (1980). *The Atman project: A transpersonal view of human development.* Wheaton, IL: Theosophical Publishing House.

Wilber, K. (1986). The spectrum of development. In K. Wilber, J. Engler, & D. P. Brown (Eds.), *Transformations of consciousness* (pp. 65–105). Boston: Shambala.

16 *Theories Focusing on the Nurse–Patient Relationship*

All theories must deal with nurse–patient relationships in some fashion, but several classes of theories take the *interchange* as their focus. This chapter looks at two sorts, the first group, interaction theories, and the second, those with an existential base.

INTERACTION THEORIES

Any theory that locates its principles in the nature of the exchange between the patient and the nurse is an interaction theory. Although these theories share a focus on the relationship itself, they vary greatly in other ways. Take, for example, the radical difference between Orlando (1990) and Watson (1988)—Orlando, pragmatic, tied to what is observed and what it means, Watson, metaphysical, developmental, spiritual. Yet both theories rest their principles on the interplay between the two actors: patient and nurse.

Interaction Communications Models

Orlando's theory is interactional because it depends on a ritualized dance, back and forth, between patient and nurse—a dance in which each party has an assigned role. The nurse observes the patient's behavior, interprets it, then reflects back to the patient what she has seen and what she thinks it means. The patient, in turn, reflects on the behavior, correcting errors, if any, in her interpretation, often gaining insight into behaviors not previously brought to the forefront of his attention. Only after the nurse knows the meaning of the behavior as the patient sees it, does she act on the behavior to solve the patient's problem. As Orlando (1990) says:

> *Learning how to understand what is happening between herself and the patient is the central core of the nurse's practice and comprises the basic framework for the help she gives to patients. (p. 5)*

As an interaction theory, Orlando locates nursing in communication—verbal and behavioral—as do most early interaction theories. The vulnerability of these theories is that they are hard to apply to patients who cannot communicate (the unconscious, confused, or withdrawn).

King's (1990) theory is another dance of roles between patient and nurse. Her theory is built on a communications model in which patient and nurse mutually perceive, judge, act, react, interact, then mutually transact. As King (1990) describes it:

> *All behavior is communication that can be observed directly or indirectly. Experiences can be communicated from one person to another to build a common frame of reference. This can be called a reciprocally contingent interaction, which means that the behavior of patients is influenced by the behavior of nurses and vice versa. Transactions occur within systems of interactions of person with person, person with object, in which continuous motion and energy exchange is organized by information. When there is a disturbance in patterns of transactions, something has disrupted abilities to function, and individuals seek assistance. (p. 83)*
>
> *Interactions are reciprocal. When one initiates an interaction with another, an action takes place, then each person reacts to the other, and a reciprocal spiral develops in which the individuals continue to interact or withdraw from the situation. Each has something to give to the other that the other wants or needs, which may be facilitated by active participation of both individuals in the situation. There is a mutuality, an interdependence in the situation in which both achieve goals. (p. 84)*

Both Orlando and King are vulnerable to the question of boundary, that is, they need to explain what context makes the interaction a *nursing* interaction as opposed to an interaction of another kind. Peplau, another nurse theorist with an interaction theory, escapes this criticism by closely tying her mid-range theory to psychiatric nursing or psychotherapeutics in nursing. Peplau, whose works have been gathered and edited by O'Toole and Welt (1989), has a goal-directed theory whose aim is to "help move the patient in a direction favoring productive social living outside of the hospital" (p. 197). She describes a patient's goal perception in the following manner:

Psychiatric patients are embarked on a search for truth about themselves and their life experiences. This search is not for the literal, factual truths but rather for the inner truths about their perceptions and attributions of their experiences and the consequences in relationships with people. (O'Toole & Welt, p. 275)

Peplau identifies the human flaw (in the patient) that makes her interpersonal relation unidirectional (unlike King who stresses reciprocity). For Peplau, the nurse is in command and sees it as her job not to let the conversation degenerate into social chit-chat. However, the method of conversation intimately involves both players. As Peplau (O'Toole & Welt, 1989) says:

Psychiatric patients are lacking the intellectual and interpersonal competencies so necessary for the work involved in their search for self-understanding. It is the quality of the verbal participation of nurses in their interactions with patients—listening and posing investigative questions—that slowly but surely stimulates the development of these competencies in patients. (p. 275)

Peplau's nurse is an investigator, prober, interpreter, and reporter, using the rich data she extracts from the patient concerning his life. She develops insight (hers and his) into the meaning of a patient's behavior (including verbal behavior) and helps the patient recognize and change patterns that obstruct achievement of his goals. Not that Peplau comes right out and says this in her writings. Instead, she reveals her principles in demonstration, showing her process in individual cases that illustrate the effective nurse. She keeps her cases related to psychiatric (or psychological) nursing, for example, nurse responses to unique patient cases of anxiety, frustration, withdrawal, loneliness, and aggression. Use of the case method allows her reader to gain insights through the "aha" method, a teaching technique that is often thought superior to merely spelling out one's principles.

All three authors, Orlando, King, and Peplau, have a *process* of interaction. Although Orlando and King apply theirs to situations in which nurses and patients meet, the content and context elements of their theories are not tightly defined or delimited. Without this work, it is difficult to say nonnurses could not use the same process. Peplau, on the other hand, has content and context pieces—phenomena located in psychiatric nursing.

Interaction Models in New Paradigm Theories

Although the content and context of new paradigm models have little in common with the interaction theories just discussed, they share the focus on the unique nurse–patient interrelationship. Watson's (1988) theory asserts that "caring as an intersubjective human process is the moral ideal of nursing" (p. 39). She explains:

> *The human care transactions provide a coming together and establish-*
> *ment of contact between persons; one's mind–body–soul engages with*
> *another's mind–body–soul in a lived moment. The shared moment of the*
> *present has the potential to transcend time and space and the physical,*
> *concrete world as we generally view it in the traditional nurse–patient*
> *relationship. (p. 47)*

Although the prior interaction theories envisioned a phenomenal nurse–patient relationship, Watson's theory envisions, instead, a transcendental one, a relationship "with the potential to transcend time and space"—nothing down to earth here. Depending on one's personal perspective, Watson's theory makes the others sound old-fashioned, or, conversely, the others make hers sound frivolous and unrealistic. These two perspectives illustrate the point that external criticism (how well a theory reflects the reality) is in the mind of the beholder.

EXISTENTIAL THEORIES

The next type of theory to focus on the nurse–patient relationship is the existential theory. Earlier, an existential interpretation was described as one in which the human agent's acts, ideas, or impulses are what characterizes the world. Within that interpretation, a whole school of philosophy, existentialism, emerged and held sway in the philosophical and public press over three decades ago. Nursing also had its existential advocates. The theorists most known for expressing this position are Paterson and Zderad. They are included here because, even today, some nurses follow their theory. More commonly, elements of it are borrowed and tucked into other theories—often the emerging New Age developmental ones. To understand what is unique about their theory, we will review the basic themes and drives in existentialism.

Dominant Themes in Existentialism

In existentialism, one begins with what exists—in this case, the human agent. (I lean heavily on the German existentialists for the interpretation that follows.) Existence precedes essence: the agent exists but what he becomes is not predetermined. There is no foreor-dained human nature. Man exists; his *being there* is the first reality about him. He is, as Heidegger (1962, pp. 78–90) says, thrown into the world. The existentialist starts with absurdity—that man simply is there (an absurdity because it does not relate to some other cause or explanation).

Furthermore, man is the only being who asks why he is there. A dog lives out his life without ever asking why he exists—but not man. Introspection, then, characterizes man; he not only exists but asks what it *means* to exist. He is concerned with the fact of his own existence.

Another tenet of existentialism is that, once he exists, man creates himself, that is, determines his own essence. The freedom to create, to choose, is one of the major themes of existentialism. One chooses, and what one chooses determines what one becomes. One literally makes himself through his choices. Because choosing is an ongoing necessity, man is never a finished product; he is always in the state of becoming. Although existentialism escapes the fatalism of a deterministic philosophy (where every act is preordained by what preceded it), the freedom it espouses is not without its price. The existentialist cannot blame today's bad choice on yesterday's events; he is fully responsible for each choice he makes. Although the past is determined (it cannot be changed), the future is open to any possibility (Sartre, 1965, pp. 409–532). Hence time is experienced as "the present toward the future."

To choose is a freedom that some perceive as a burden. Some choices, for example, must be made over and over again. A dieter decides anew every time he passes the refrigerator. A marriage vow must be confirmed again every time an opportunity to negate it arises. The need to decide in the ongoing present (and the responsibility for the decision) are central themes in existentialism. Choices once made are irrevocable; one cannot turn back the clock to undo a decision. One cannot ever again be the person he was before a particular decision was made. The past is fixed, and he is responsible for it. The future is open to whatever choices he makes.

Nor is it possible to choose with knowledge. One cannot debate: if I make Choice X, I will become this type of person, but if I make Choice Y, I will become that sort. Decision-making is not grounded in knowledge. On the contrary, knowledge is the result of decision-making and subsequent action. It is not possible to predict with certainty; so one makes choices and thereby chooses oneself without knowing what the result will be.

The need to choose in the light of uncertainty calls for a leap into the unknown, and for this reason many existentialists associate choice with dread, anxiety, or despair (Kierkegaard, 1954, pp. 147–207). Other philosophers delight in the creativity and power of such ultimate freedom, celebrating, instead of dreading, those leaps into the unknown. Because *choice* is what constitutes man, to choose in light of the unknown represents an authentic, honest mode of being. Avoidance of choice and escapism of various sorts represent inauthentic modes of being—being as *nonbeing*. Nonbeing is an alienation from oneself; authenticity is a major virtue.

Failure to accept responsibility for the results of one's choices is also *inauthentic* being. One acts and is accountable. Denial of one's emotions is another form of inauthenticity; to negate one's feelings is dishonest because it denies one's experiences.

The existential philosophy has little room for intentions; what counts is acts performed, not acts—or results—intended. One is what one does; acts define the self. Potentialities do not count. Because the results of leaps into the unknown, occasioned by choices, cannot be predicted rationally, the existential philosophy is based on examination of passions rather than reason. Feeling is concrete, particular, immediate, and subjective; in contrast, thinking is universal, abstract, removed from immediacy, and objective. Suffering often is posited as the origin of consciousness in existentialism. Awareness of self does not arise through thought. Theories do not give us reality; reality must be experienced.

Many (but not all) philosophers who are classified as existentialists share these dominant themes:

1. Man exists as being in the world, and his existence precedes his essence (what he becomes).
2. Freedom and choice characterize man.
3. Man forms himself through his choices.
4. Freedom may be seen as terrible and burdensome or as a joy.
5. Emotion and passion characterize man better than does reason.
6. The individual (not the society or group) is the proper unit of analysis.

Nature of the Self in Existentialism

In existentialism, the quest is for understanding of the self and what it means to be a human. Many writers propose that a self has the following characteristics:

1. The self feels unfinished, incomplete; he exists as an open being, always becoming, never finished.
2. The self does not experience a mind–body split but feels himself to be a whole.
3. The self perceives himself as a unity, despite the fact that

he has many selves in that he fills many different roles in his day-to-day life.

4. Although he may change radically over time, man perceives himself as an ongoing unity; he has a sense of a continuing *me*.

5. The nature of that *me*, extracted from the content with which it deals, is problematic; motion or drive may be its chief characteristic.

The search for understanding of self (that which is conscious of its own being) is critical in existential thought. The source of knowledge is a close examination of one's own feelings, responses, and awareness of being. Evidence is not of the analytical sort found in scientific research.

Existential Relationships

Existentialists differ on the nature of the relationship between self and other. Some claim that only knowledge of the self is possible, that the other is merely an object for the self. Other theorists argue that if one accepts the reality of being for oneself, then one must grant it for others.

Many existentialists focus on man's intersubjectivity, exploring the nature of *genuine encounter*. (This is where the existential philosophy enters into the theories based on the nurse–patient relationship.) Typically, an authentic encounter is seen as one in which each person reveals his authentic being to the other and in which each person is able to grasp the reality of the other person.

Existential Applications in Nursing

The initial attraction of existentialism for nurses is accounted for by the apparent fit of the existential reality with the nursing environment. Because authentic relationships occur one-to-one, the format is natural for nursing. Further, the nurse finds herself in an environment in which she (and the dyadic other) are exposed to strong emotions, questions concerning self-worth, and even fears for the continued existence of the self. Moreover, the situation demands that the nurse face constant choices (often critical) in providing care, as does the patient concerning his welfare.

Sister Vaillot (1962) describes the existential environment in relation to student nurses:

> They see people grieve, suffer, or rejoice with an intensity that seems hardly possible for humans to bear. They see women give birth, and

they see patients die. They see men and women in such crises that they are stripped naked of what they have: wealth, prestige, beauty, status, intelligence, and only the person that they really are is left. Student nurses are, almost every minute of their professional life, confronted with the choice between acceptance and refusal of these situation-limits. They can be a presence to patients, and follow the road leading to authentic being. (p. 42)

Vaillot, like other existentialists, focuses on commitment, not knowledge. Jourard (1971) stays in the emotive vein but focuses on the evolving self of the nurse as it relates to potentiality for nursing others:

The becoming general nursing practitioner is a person who is open to her own experience, who genuinely cares about people and about herself. This is important. She cares about herself. The proof of effective caring about oneself is a self which is happy, growing, open. (p. 284)

Jourard contrasts this sort of personal growth and becoming with education, efficiency, and effortlessness, asserting that these traits (often associated with professionalism) may actively obstruct growth (p. 285). Again the existential focus is on authenticity, not cognition.

Sarosi (1968) also describes nursing in existential terms:

Nursing action, then, is affirmation and validation of human experience, and is characterized by involvement, not composure or "objectivity." The desired outcome is wholeness, not comfort. (p. 353)

Realization of uniqueness, of human finiteness, may be experienced by the individual through his encounter with death and loneliness. Thus loneliness and death must be confronted rather than escaped from. It is this encounter which leads man to the infinite, to an awareness of "the inseparability of his organism from the cosmos. Existence is relationship; to be is to be related." (p. 356)

The classic existential nurse theorists are Paterson and Zderad (1988); the flavor of their work together can be sensed in the following quotations:

Nurses experience with other human beings peak life events: creation, birth, winning, nothingness, losing, separation, death. . . . Through intouchness with self, authentic awareness and reflection on such experiences the human nurse comes to know. Humanistic nursing practice theory asks that the nurse describe what she comes to know: (1) the nurse's unique perspective and responses, (2) the other's knowable responses, and (3) the reciprocal call and response, the between, as they occur in the nursing situation. (pp. 6–7)

The focus is on awareness, authenticity, and on the emotional, experiential aspects of nursing. The next quotation not only reveals their existential base but shows why existential nursing theories find their principle in relationships:

> *In real life, nursing phenomena may be experienced from the reference points of nurturing, of being nurtured, or of the nurturing process in the "between." For instance, the nurse may describe comfort as an experience of comforting another person; the patient, as an experience of being comforted. However, while each has experienced something within himself, he also has experienced something of the "between," namely the message of meaning of the "comforting-being comforted" process. This essential interhuman dimension of nursing is beyond and yet within the technical, procedural, or interactional elements of the event. It is a quality of being that is expressed in the doing. (p. 13)*

This older existentialist language resembles the language of some theorists in the New Age paradigm. The themes sound similar, but the context is different. Existentialists deal with phenomenal experience—what is seen, felt—directly. In contrast, the New Agers seek transcendental explanations for events, in phenomena like energy exchanges, resonating waves, human fields. Although there are religious existentialists, they are usually in mainstream religious orthodoxy. In contrast, the New Agers express man's spirituality as a development toward higher levels of being or in which man participates in an ultimate conscious unity. Despite these differences, the flavor of these two movements (existentialism and New Ageism) is similar, particularly the great human sensitivity for the other and the self. Both of these nursing philosophies focus on the one-to-one human relationship as the vehicle through which nursing takes place.

The nurse theorist who advocates an existential approach must ask serious questions concerning the nature of nursing. If an existential interpretation is merely an overlay, not actually affecting what the nurse does, then it is not an inherent part of a nursing theory. It is not enough to advocate an existential approach in nursing; one must say how it changes the day-to-day acts of nurses. When an existential approach is used to explain nurse behavior that could occur under any other nursing philosophy, then the application is superficial. The existential goal (authentic being), for example, may be incompatible with some well accepted, traditional nursing goals. Does the nurse remain true to the existential values despite the professional norms?

The approach to the patient in pain illustrates the potential conflict. From an existential viewpoint, suffering serves to bring about a state of self-awareness, thereby creating an openness to authentic experience. Suffering brings a person face to face with his own being. Yet most nurses would seek to alleviate suffering rather than prolong it as an instrument of self-realization. A nurse who purports to use an existential theory must be prepared to deal with challenges such as this.

Similarly, the skills of communication taught to nurses often are manipulative devices designed to achieve certain ends—possibly worthy ends—but not the end of genuine intersubjectivity. The issue of manipulation (inauthentic being—treating the other as an object) must be addressed in a truly existential nursing theory. Then there is the issue of genuine encounter. Most existentialists consider genuine encounter to be an experience that shakes one's self-world. Hence, one need ask how many such encounters a nurse could be expected to endure. A nurse–patient relationship arises in every patient care assignment, but can genuine encounters be assigned? Furthermore genuine encounters are *two-way* interactions, and some patients may not wish to play the game.

One might argue that in an era when so many illnesses are related to life-style, an existential approach holds interesting promise, and it is used today in some substance abuse programs. Unlike the Alcoholic Anonymous programs that treat alcoholism as a disease, confrontational programs administer a reality shock by placing blame and challenging the alcoholic to accept responsibility for his own conduct. The Toughlove program for parents of substance-abusing youths has a confrontational theme.

Existential theories of nursing, best represented by Paterson and Zderad, appear to have been upstaged by theories focused in a New Age paradigm. Yet one sees some similarities. Compare, for example, Paterson and Zderad's (1988, pp. 27–29) notion of the nurse as *presence* with Quinn's (1992) notion of the nurse as a sacred place, a healing environment.

Parse (1981) is a good example of the crossover from existentialism to New Ageism. Indeed, one could argue that she still sits on the fence between the two ideologies. Take her assumptions, which she admittedly draws from Heidegger (1962), Merleau-Ponty (1962, 1963), and Sartre (1957, 1965), (all existentialists) as well as from Rogers (1970), whose work was instrumental in initiating New Ageism in nursing. Parse's (1981) assumptions—rearranged for this purpose—include but are not limited to:

- *Man is an open being, freely choosing meaning in situations, bearing responsibility for decisions.*
- *Health is an open process of becoming, experienced by man.*
- *Man is transcending multidimensionality with the possibles.*
- *Health is unitary man's negentropic unfolding (p. 25).*

If the first two assumptions smack of existentialism, the latter two are soundly grounded in the New Age paradigm.

It may be the fact that existential and New Age philosophies both focus on the nurse–patient interrelationship that makes them bedfellows. They share a poetry of tone and sentiment that is not found in the interaction theories of King, Peplau, and Orlando, for example. Yet there is a great difference between an existentialist and an advocate of a New Age paradigm. Many existentialists accept the absurdity of man's existence, whereas the New Agers do not find it absurd or pointless at all.

SUMMARY

Several types of nursing theory revolve around the nurse–patient interaction. Often this is the only similarity they bear. Older interactions models tend to focus on a communications model that is based heavily on interpersonal communication. King, Peplau, and Orlando represent this trend. Their age is not the measure of their use in the profession, and all three models are still used today. Newer interaction models occur in the New Age paradigm, but here the notion of communication has expanded to encompass much more than verbal communication. Notions of mind–body–soul engagement between patient and nurse illustrate these larger notions of communication.

Existential theories of authentic encounter also are found under the category of nurse–patient interaction. These older theories often have been replaced by New Age paradigm images or melded with ideas arising in this new context. Whatever the source, theories based on the nurse–patient interaction place their principles in the critical juncture between two people rather than in one or the other.

REFERENCES

Heidegger, M. (1962). *Being and time.* (J. Macquarrie & E. Robinson, Trans.). New York: Harper & Row.

Jourard, S. (1971). *The transparent self.* New York: Van Nostrand Reinhold.

Kierkegaard, S. (1954). *The sickness unto death.* (W. Lowrie, Trans.). Garden City, NY: Doubleday.

King, I. (1990). King's conceptual framework and theory of goal attainment. In M. E. Parker (Ed.), *Nursing theories in practice* (pp. 73–84). New York: National League for Nursing Press.

Merleau-Ponty, M. (1962). *Phenomenology of perception.* New York: Humanities Press.

Merleau-Ponty, M. (1963). *The structure of behavior.* Boston: Beacon Press.

Orlando, I. J. (1990). *The dynamic nurse-patient relationship.* New York: National League for Nursing Press.

O'Toole, A. W., & Welt, S. R. (Eds.). (1989). *Interpersonal theory in nursing practice: Selected works of Hildegard E. Peplau.* New York: Springer.

Parse, R. R. (1981). *Man-living-health: A theory of nursing.* New York: Wiley.

Paterson, J. G., & Zderad, L. T. (1988). *Humanistic nursing.* New York: National League for Nursing Press.

Quinn, J. F. (1992, July). Holding sacred space: The nurse as healing environment. *Holistic Nursing Practice, 4,* 26–36.

Rogers, M. E. (1970). *An introduction to the theoretical basis of nursing.* Philadelphia: Davis.

Sarosi, G. M. (1968). A critical theory: The nurse as a fully human person. *Nursing Forum, 4,* 349–364.

Sartre, J. P. (1957). *Transcendence of the ego.* New York: Noonday Press.

Sartre, J. P. (1965). *Being and nothingness.* (H. E. Barnes, Trans.). New York: Citadel Press.

Vaillot, M. C. (1962). *Commitment to nursing: A philosophic investigation.* Philadelphia: Lippincott.

Watson, J. (1988). *Nursing: Human science and human care: A theory of nursing.* New York: National League for Nursing Press.

17 Resource-Driven Nursing: A Model for Practice and Management

PRACTICE MODELS

Nurses have had to adjust to increasingly difficult work situations. In many cases, they have had to lower their expectations concerning what could be accomplished for patients. An adjustment to scarcities in nursing staff, in proper supplies and equipment, and in support staff, despite increasing patient acuity, has been the rule, not the exception. Many nurses are dissatisfied with their roles, not to mention disillusioned with the health care system. Nowhere has the difference between expectations and realities been greater than in the acute care facility. We will use this setting for the following discussion although the principles derived can be applied in any setting in today's progressive "pass down" tactics.

Total Patient Care

A generation of nurses was educated on the model that preceded resource-driven care, that is, total patient care (comprehensive nursing care). This system assumed that the nurse would provide "everything" for the patients assigned to her. There was no notion of compromise, of limitations, no sense that a patient was only paying for X amount of care.

The model of total patient care worked well in ideal conditions, but a model made for ideal conditions is vulnerable where nurses cannot produce those conditions. That is what happened; conditions changed, yet many nurses still hold themselves accountable for standards they cannot achieve. Worse, these nurses place their notion of self-worth in the comprehensiveness of their care for each patient. If they cannot do "everything" needed, they judge themselves to be failures.

The concept of *total patient care* was based on idealistic goals set in the abstract. No constraints were to be considered; the nurse was limited in identifying patient needs only by her own intellectual capacities. She was responsible for providing everything that was deemed to be good for the patient. In this respect, total patient care was a *goal-driven* model (Barnum & Kerfoot, 1995, pp. 10–14). A nurse could not claim success unless she identified all the potential patient needs, set all the possible goals, and met them.

In recent years, total nursing care (goal-driven care) has been a memory in many places as nurses have been forced to compromise with their ideals. A makeshift sort of care evolved, a care pattern that might be called *doing what one could*. This is a case in which a practice arose before it was framed in theoretical terms. This chapter provides a theoretical structure that both reflects the practice (doing what one could) and sets forth the dimensions of a model so that nurses function effectively in the system rather than fumbling through without a plan.

The Resource-Driven Model

In contrast to goal-driven care, today's care should be labeled *re-source-driven care*. In a resource-driven model, the nurse first considers her environment and the resources it holds. Only then does she determine what goals she reasonably can take on for a patient or a group of patients. The resources drive the goals, not the other way around. This is the opposite of the total patient care concept, where goals are set first, assuming that the necessary resources will be found.

Resource-driven care stands the old model on its head, and that hits hard at a philosophy of care most nurses hold dear. It is particularly hard for a nurse who has been indoctrinated to think that her worth is tied to doing "everything" for her patients. It calls for a new outlook, a new measure with which to gauge one's worth.

A resource-driven model also is more complex than a goal-driven model. It demands more choices, a more accurate fit between available resources and the work to be done. If total patient care took its origin in quality factors of good care, then resource-driven care demands a mesh of quality and quantity (how much care at what quality).

The most important quantity factor in the new system is the nurse's own work time. The question becomes how much and what sort of care she can deliver in a limited number of hours. Other resources may expand, but one never gets more than 24 hours in a day. True, a nurse may compensate by working overtime (usually without pay), but she will find that she can only subsidize the system so long before she is mentally and physically bankrupt.

In their school days, nurses could take hours in the library to complete a single nursing care plan. The nurse did not have to make hard choices; she poured everything into that care plan, being careful not to skip a single goal that might help the patient. Resource-driven care does not have that luxury. Today's nurse must balance the needs of a group of patients who typically have more conjoined needs than can possibly be tackled. She must make complex professional decisions—determining what things she will do for which patients, knowing that her priorities are critical, and that she must often choose between the essential and the merely beneficial. Indeed, the resource-driven model is a triage model not unlike that used in emergency room or disaster nursing.

COMPARISON OF SYSTEMS

There are numerous dimensions on which the resource-driven and goal-driven models differ. The first has to do with underlying assumptions. For the goal-driven model, it was assumed that all worthy goals would be tackled. With initiative, the nurse would find the necessary resources, including the requisite time. The resource-driven model has no such optimism. It assumes that the nurse's time is finite and so is her access to additional resources. She must plan within the constraints of accessible manpower, supplies, and equipment available in the institution. These items are unlikely to expand simply because she identifies a need for them.

If a nurse fails to understand the environment in which she is working, she is at a great disadvantage for achieving her goals. Simply, she will have the wrong goals for the wrong time. They will not be goals that interest others, especially those who have more power in the system.

Some nurses take a rigid position that a failure to do "everything" for one's patients implies a nursing fault. Kritek (1995, pp. 207–236), in contrast, directs us to recognize accurately our level of power in negotiating within the health care system. She also directs us to use that power to optimize and enhance our influence. First, we must have a realistic view of our power:

> *Uneven tables are negotiation situations in which there is a structured and unacknowledged inequity among the participants. At such tables, participants assume that the inequity will continue to be unacknowledged and perpetuated. Thus, the negotiations are tainted before they begin. Outcomes of such a negotiation preserve at least one dimension of the conflict while purportedly attempting to address another.* (p. 228)

In a situation calling for resource-driven care, the nurse who attempts to deliver comprehensive care is at a great disadvantage. She has lost what negotiating power she had because she does not negotiate concerning goals that have meaning to others in the organization. The first difference between the two systems (goal-driven and resource-driven), then, is that they tend to mediate different values.

The process of planning patient care also is different in the two models. In the goal-driven model, the nurse sets goals based on the patient's case description or her own assessments. When she has set all the desirable goals she can determine, she decides on the methods (interventions) to achieve the goals. Next, she implements the methods. Finally, she evaluates whether or not the goals have been achieved. The process in the resource-driven model is more complex, beginning, not with an assessment of the patient, but with an assessment of the resources at hand. How many hours will she work? What staff, if any, are assigned to assist her? What sorts of supports are available? Whereas the goal-directed nurse begins with a quality issue (the patient's needs and goals), the resource-directed nurse starts with a quantity assessment of resources—man-hours available being the most important single calculation.

The resource-directed nurse then assesses the patient(s) as to needs and calculates potential goals for care. One patient's care cannot be calculated alone, unless he comprises the nurse's full assignment. Instead, she considers as a whole the needs and potential goals for a case load of patients. Next, she prioritizes, deciding what *must* be done, what is less critical. She works with a realization that not "everything" is likely to be achieved. She matches her priorities to the available resources.

Concerning her chief resource, her own time, the nurse cannot go directly from prioritized goals to an estimation of time required because the time required may depend on the methods she selects to meet those goals. The interim step requires that goals be considered in relation to alternate means of achieving them. For many goals, there may be some methods that are preferred (in the abstract), others that may be less adequate but take less time and fewer resources. A subtle dance of professional judgment takes place. What goals can she meet, using what methods, all within the constraints of her resources? It was much simpler for the goal-directed nurse who could do "everything" and did not have to make any hard choices. The nurse using the resource-driven model must be a more competent professional to make the best calculations. In this situation, the nurse who says, "I was too busy to practice professionally today," misses the whole point. Hard choices call for sophisticated professional decisions.

The evaluation process is more complex in the resource-driven model. The nurse using a goal-driven model need only ask if she had achieved her goals. The nurse using the resource-driven model must make many more judgments:

1. Did she make an *accurate* assessment of resources? Were there resources available that she failed to consider? Did she overestimate her available time, for example, or the assistance she could call on from a helper?
2. Did she take on an appropriate *number* of goals? Did she bite off too much, too little?
3. Did she take on the *most important* goals? Or did she skip something that should have had a higher priority? Did she waste time on some goals that were impossible to achieve?
4. Did she choose the best methods, considering the circumstances? Were there more efficient systems available? Were the methods effective?
5. Did she achieve the goals selected? In this last element, she comes back to the only evaluation item required on the goal-driven system.

LIMITATIONS AND ADVANTAGES OF BOTH SYSTEMS

The limitation of the goal-driven system is that it breaks down if the assumed resources cannot be found. For example, if the nurse does not have the time she anticipates, then not all her goals are achieved. Worse, because she may not realize the deficit until well into her work shift, the things that get done and the things that get omitted may be unrelated to their importance. Finally, if the goal-driven system lacks the anticipated resources, the nurse has no recourse but to feel like a failure.

The resource-driven model has its limitations too. First, it calls for more sophisticated practice if the right decisions are to be made. Additionally, the resource-driven model requires a safety net. That means criteria must be set for recognizing when scarce resources are reaching the level of unsafe care. This is done by setting nursing standards and identifying indices that will quickly signal a dangerous situation. In simple terms, one index might be that of the lowest acceptable nurse–patient ratio. Criteria for recognizing a critical situation and plans for how to deal with the contingency should be set *in advance* of such a situation occurring.

What are the advantages of each system? The goal-driven system has the charm of allowing the nurse to practice at the peak of her performance, while assuring the patient of the best possible outcomes. Further, the nursing process and its evaluation are comparatively simple, allowing less experienced nurses to achieve success with minimal stress. In contrast, the resource-driven model has the advantage of adapting to its environment when it is not within the nurse's power to change it. In a resource-scarce environment, this can be a distinct advantage. Further, a nurse working in such circumstance can still feel satisfied with her performance. She can say to herself, "Given the circumstances, I made the best choices possible, did the most and most effective work that could be done." The resource-driven model also works in a resource-rich environment. When the nurse calculates what can be done in this case, she will find herself able to take on a plethora of goals.

RELATIONSHIP TO CASE MANAGEMENT AND MANAGED CARE

Complementary systems management structures have arisen that structure the work of nurses using a resource-driven model. Case management care trajectories spell out the specific care that should be delivered to a patient with a given condition, within a given time frame (Cohen & Cesta, 1997). This standardization streamlines care, selecting for the nurse the priorities to be achieved. Further, the procedures are tightly associated with expected patient outcomes to ensure a given level of success. At the same time, managed care and its control of reimbursement ensure that additional costly efforts will not be pursued or at least will not be reimbursed.

Altogether, the system of resource-driven care, combined with managed care and case management, creates an intricate web of mutually controlled relationships in a logistic pattern of interacting components. The system is highly programmed, highly complex, goal directed (by outcomes), and guided by predetermined relationships between the nursing processes and patient outcomes. In most systems today, the case management aspect incorporates other professionals, along with nurses, in the case plan.

ADDITIONAL THOUGHTS

Advocates of the resource-driven model would assert that excellence in nursing practice has never truly been separate from environmental conditions. Excellent nursing, such advocates would say, can occur in the most difficult of circumstances. Nightingale started a profession in Crimea despite her bleak surroundings (because of her bleak surroundings, some would say). Excellence is optimizing on the possible; simply put, it is what one does with what one has. The question is one of the nurse's assumed power to change an environment. The goal-driven model assumes she can do so to an extent encompassing the best of all worlds. The resource-driven model is more realistic, recognizing that not all of the negative factors within the environment are within her control, certainly not in today's care arena. The resource-driven model asks how well the nurse did in the circumstance, not how well she did in the abstract. Nurses educated on a model of the ideal may not be comfortable with this model initially, but it builds a new standard for judging one's worth.

MANAGEMENT MODELS

In basic management models, we find a situation that corresponds directly to the care delivery models. Just as a resource-driven model has replaced goal-driven nursing care, so a resource-driven model has replaced a goal-driven model in management. The older management by objectives (MBO) is clearly a goal-driven model—just look at its name. The pattern is identical to goal-driven nursing care: first you set the goals, then you find the resources.

Strategic Management

Management by objectives has been replaced by a strategic management model (Barnum & Mallard, 1989, pp. 66–69) that, like resource-driven nursing, starts by assessing the environment—internal to the organization and external to it. Strategic management assesses the organization's strengths and weaknesses in comparison to those of the competition. This marketplace mentality, tied as it is to environmental conditions, makes strategic management and the resource-driven care model parallel ideologies.

Only after the environment is carefully scanned and assessed will goals be selected in the strategic management model. Goals will be those that can reasonably be taken on given environmental constraints, or those that optimize on opportunities. As with the resource-driven model, the focus is on picking and choosing the right actions. The effective organization is the one that makes the most advantageous choices, based on the most accurate assessment of the environment.

In strategic planning, the management scheme is designed with the environment in mind and is made flexible to change as the external environment changes. Quick response is more important than the old 2-year and 5-year plans of MBO. Assessment, of necessity, becomes ongoing rather than periodic. In strategic management the image is moving, swift, changing—not like MBO where one assumed that most elements were in one's control. In strategic planning, like the resource-driven care model, the outside world impinges on and affects one's plans.

Strategic planning involves drawing up alternate scenarios, alternate plans designed for meeting different environmental contingencies. The strategic plan lacks the stability and security of the MBO model; it is not a simple rational plan. The vulnerability of MBO is its assumption that one *can* plan ahead. It assumes a stable world, where one can set goals that will be appropriate 1, 2, or 5 years later. In a world changing as fast as today's health care, such an assumption will not work.

Management Models

Mintzberg (1973) anticipated the changing models of management over two decades ago when he wrote about three managerial styles: the rational planning, adaptive, and entrepreneurial modes. His rational planning model sounded perfect then; it typified the MBO approach where all planning was done in advance. The system seemed ideal in a world where effects of actions could be predicted and anticipated to hold over long time spans. Nurses wrote in praise of the model then, not inaccurately labeling it proactive instead of reactive.

From today's perspective, however, the other two models make more sense. The entrepreneurial mode allows the risk taker, who has just a bit more vision or predictive power than the rest, to make her mark in an uncertain world. She takes bold strokes—and wins or loses accordingly. This form of management has great possibilities in a world where unexpected changes can happen overnight. The environment is indeed ripe for the ambitious, clever entrepreneur.

However, most health care management presently focuses on the adaptive model instead of the entrepreneurial model. The shifting environment makes adaptation challenge enough for any manager. Strategic planning epitomizes this view with its constant reassessment of the environment and its rapid response to changes.

Strategic management is not the only new model around. In

nursing management, as in other management systems, one sees the adoption of *futures management*, an ideology that tries to have the best of both the goal-driven and resource-driven models. Preferred futures management, like strategic planning, envisions various future scenarios. Then, like the goal-driven model, it selects the preferred scenario (setting goals, in other words).

Then the model switches back to the action-oriented strategic management approach—or better yet, to the entrepreneurial model— for the manager takes the bold strides to try to bring about that preferred future (Anvaripour, Bezold, & Weissman, 1990). Choosing a preferred future and making it happen is quite different from the *forecasting* advocated in the MBO model. In the MBO notion, the future was externally imposed; one strove to predict it, not create it.

Like Mintzberg, Drucker builds management models that reflect today's era. Drucker's (1995) four basic principles for a theory of business apply easily to nursing and health care management. He identifies three essential components to be assessed: the environment, the mission, and the core competencies of the business. Concerning these aspects, he says:

1. *The assumptions about environment, mission, and core competencies must fit reality.*
2. *The assumptions in all three areas have to fit one another.*
3. *The theory of the business must be known and understood throughout the organization.*
4. *The theory of the business has to be tested constantly. (pp. 30–31)*

Here, again, we see the influence of environment and its fit with the organization's mission and abilities.

LEADERSHIP AND THE TRANSFORMATIONAL LEADER

Not only do the new management models reflect the nature of the times, so do the images of the manager. In the era of MBO, the leader was contrasted with the manager, and the manager usually came out ahead. One could be educated to be a manager; the process was definitive and logical. This training process was more to be desired than spontaneous and undisciplined leadership.

Now, in an era when the future is difficult to predict and the environment is characterized by frequent, unpredictable changes, the notion of leadership once again has superseded the notion of the rational manager. Transformational leadership is advocated as today's solution. The new focus is switched from what the leader *does* to who the leader *is* and how she motivates those who are led.

Unlike the prior management ideology, transformational leadership assumes that the leader and followers have the same purpose and that they can raise one another to higher levels of motivation and morality. This notion certainly has appeal where both leader and followers are professionals.

The notion of transformational leadership is often tied to the New Age paradigm (Barker, 1991). Barker asserts that a new view of humanness is emerging, that people bring to the workplace a new set of beliefs and values. The old paradigm, in contrast, focused on logical decision-making and rationality.

Transformational leadership is more human, with the leader seeking a new set of values emerging between herself and her workers: mutual cooperation instead of competition, attention to human needs and feelings, consultative interactions instead of downward-directed orders from the hierarchy, and an empowering of all employees, not just the chief. Transformational leaders, so goes the theory, mobilize others; they grow and develop together with their followers. As one set of needs and values are satisfied for all parties, new ones surface and contribute to personal and professional growth.

The results of transformational leadership show in a focus on goals, joy in work, enthusiasm about patients and the care they receive, and a sense of accomplishment shared by all. These characteristics differ from the sort of talk one hears under an MBO ideology, that is, quotas, specified outcomes, measurements, data—cold, hard, incontrovertible facts.

The strategies used by a transformational leader, paraphrased from Barker (1991, pp. 206–207), involve:

- Creating a vision
- Building a social architecture that shows how that vision will be institutionalized
- Sustaining organizational trust
- Recognizing the importance of building self-esteem

Two polarities have always been used in looking at leadership: (1) whether the focus is on the leader or the followers, and (2) when the leader is the focus, whether the stress is on what she *does* or who she *is*. An MBO orientation focuses on what the leader does. Transformational leadership stresses who she is. Yet it also gives the followers more credence because the response of the followers is the measure of the transformational leader's effectiveness.

SUMMARY

In a world of uncertainty, scarce resources, and increased competition, it is not surprising that our theoretical models changed to reflect an altered environment. Models for health care system management, patient care delivery, nursing management, and nurse manager behavior all changed at the same time, in ways that make them more compatible with today's health care environment.

Practices often are established before the models are neatly described and labeled as theories. The logic of these present changes should give us faith in the ultimate wit and intelligence of humans—and certainly of our nurse leaders.

REFERENCES

Anvaripour, P., Bezold, C., & Weissman, G. (1990, April). A nursing department can and should plan for the future. *Nursing & Health Care, 4,* 207–209.

Barker, A. M. (1991, April). An emerging leadership pattern: Transformational leadership. *Nursing & Health Care, 4,* 204–207.

Barnum, B. S., & Kerfoot, K. M. (1995). *The nurse as executive* (4th ed.). Gaithersburg, MD: Aspen.

Barnum, B. S., & Mallard, C. O. (1989). *Essentials of nursing management: Concepts and contest of practice.* Rockville, MD: Aspen.

Cohen, E. L., & Cesta, T. G. (1997). *Nursing case management: From concept to evaluation* (2nd ed.). St. Louis: Mosby-Year Book.

Drucker, P. F. (1995). *Managing in a time of great change.* New York: Truman Talley Books/Dutton.

Kritek, P. B. (1995). Nursing: Negotiating at an uneven table. In L. J. Marcus, (Ed.), *Renegotiating health care: Resolving conflict to build collaboration* (pp. 207–236). San Francisco: Jossey-Bass.

Mintzberg, H. (1973). Strategy making in three modes. *California Management Review, 2,* 44–53.

18 Nursing Theory and Restructured Practice

Nursing theory has always affected practice assignment systems, even in eras before theory was recognized as such. But theory alone is not adequate to explain the work delegation systems; environmental circumstances also affect the choices. The present era has seen a radical change in care delivery, namely, the introduction of restructured or re-engineered nursing practice. Virtually every major health delivery institution has completed, or is presently involved in, restructuring its care delivery, and no two institutions are using just the same pattern. Driven by stringent economic pressures, hospitals are responding to the new payment systems, primarily featuring reimbursements through capitation. As Dunham-Taylor, Marquette, and Pinczuk (1996) explain:

> Increasingly, health care financing is moving in the direction where health maintenance organizations (HMOs) have led: capitation, or accepting a fixed amount of money per enrolled person per period (usually a year), and agreeing to provide some defined set of health care services to all plan members with no additional billing. (p. 26)

Capitation means the facility runs a risk of losing money if too many members of a plan are admitted. Consequently, they hope to decrease the cost of nursing, reducing the ratio of nurses to patients to hedge on fiscal vulnerability. Most institutions hope to retain quality of care while deceasing systems costs, including the cost of professional nursing staff. Nor is the pattern exclusive to nursing; other departments and services are similarly under the gun of restructuring, namely, streamlining procedures so that fewer personnel can do more, through enhanced efficiency.

Although every group of employees feels the pressure, nursing is particularly vulnerable for two reasons: (1) a high proportion of health care workers in most institutions are nurses so they have received greater departmental cutbacks, and (2) in the years just before retrenchment, nurses' salaries were increased significantly, making them a visible "target of opportunity" for reductions. In an industry where discretionary funds are highly limited, it was predictable that management, under orders to economize, would demand a decrease in professional nurse staffing numbers. We see a circle of historical effects whose results could have been predicted:

1. A shortage of nurses to meet the increasing demands of a health care industry where patients were sicker and sicker
2. Systematic enhancement (advertising) of nursing as a career choice, including increased salaries for nurses at all levels
3. A resultant oversupply of nurses
4. Subsequent financial crises calling for decreases in hiring of professional staff

The shortage that started the cycle has been solved, not by eliminating the need for nurses, but by learning to live with an unmet demand for care and by passing nursing tasks downward to less skilled workers. The shortage has been answered by eliminating professional positions from the marketplace.

NEW SYSTEMS

Restructured practice involves a careful analysis of the tasks that must be accomplished to deliver patient care and to achieve desired patient goals, along with an assessment of who is able to do the tasks. Often in looking at who can do what, new jobs are created with new constellations of skills and educational qualifications. The decisions involve looking anew at the premises of prior task assignment decisions. Typically, restructured practice involves adding one or more levels of employees to the lower end of the care personnel rung and moving tasks once seen as sacrosanct professional nursing turf down to lower level workers.

The principle underlying restructuring is that of not using "overqualified" personnel for tasks that can be achieved by lesser skilled personnel. In many instances this means creating new roles, combining tasks that may not have been previously joined, under a single job description.

Restructured or *re-engineered practice* are the terms most often used, but the linked term, *differentiated practice*, sometimes is used with the same meaning. The notion of differentiated practice was first heard from nurse educators and consisted of a demand that practice settings cease using all nurses as if they were alike. Educators wanted nurses to be used differentially, based on their educational credentials. Leaders who demanded differentiated practice envisioned that the baccalaureate nurse would have a more advanced role than nurses prepared in diploma and associate degree programs.

Ironically, restructured practice differentiates roles according to preparation—but in a downward direction. Most of the differentiation has been between nurses and less well prepared caregivers rather than between the baccalaureate prepared nurse and associate and diploma nurses. Nevertheless, from a theoretical perspective, the same principle was at work: task distribution according to one's abilities, each employee used to the peak of his capacity.

THE HISTORICAL PERSPECTIVE

One of the easiest ways to understand restructured practice as a theory is to look at its place relevant to other historical shifts in nursing assignment systems. The pattern, from the long view, is dialectic—that is, there is a clear pattern of thesis, antithesis, and synthesis. A new assignment system always arises in opposition to the system it replaces. The new system comes into being just when the flaws of the prior system have reached their peak irritation value. After an initial flurry of enthusiasm, the new pattern becomes the norm, and, in time, its own limitations become onerous. Eventually, another system comes along to challenge this one—and the pattern continues.

What brings an irritation to the forefront? In some cases it is simply the test of time. In others, the environment influencing the assignment system changes, making its flaws more visible. In the newest shift to restructured practice, an altered environment forced a new system into being. Chief among the presses was the fact that institutions could no longer afford to hire all the nurses required for patient care needs.

The history of assignment systems in the United States gives one a sense of how the shift occurred. In this nation, even nursing in hospitals, began with a *private duty* nursing model. The old private duty nurse had exclusive responsibility for planning for and doing for one patient. In this sense, private duty was a highly *patient-oriented* system. The nurse's role included around-the-clock care duties with few days off. Often the nurse slept on a cot in the patient's hospital room, not unlike the system for nursing in the home.

That pattern began to rub because of an environmental change: World War II, with nurses marching off to tend to the troops. In the subsequent civilian shortage of nurses, so-called *functional nursing* was conceived. As expected, it was the antithesis of the private duty model. Functional nursing was driven by a need to improve the efficiency, to get more mileage from the few nurses available. The essential step was to shift from a *patient-based* system to a *task-based* system by the simple expedient of giving the hospital nurse tasks rather than patients. Instead of each nurse doing everything for one patient, tasks for patients on a unit were divided up on a factory line model.

It was realized that a "medicine nurse" could distribute drugs for a whole floor of patients with greater efficiency than could 10 nurses setting up separate medication trays for their patients. The model has other specialist roles: the treatment nurse, the bedside caregiver, the temperature taker, the bedmaker, and so forth. The theory was that a worker doing a limited number of tasks would grow expert at those tasks, improving the overall system efficiency. The model achieved its goal: the greatest efficiency with the fewest workers. By dividing tasks, the model allowed for creation of subordinate workers who might do the tasks requiring the least skill.

Eventually several flaws in the functional nursing system became evident, chief among them the fact that patient needs not fitting into the role categories (medicines, treatments, baths) tended to fall through the cracks. In addition, patients suffered from personnel overload: too many people coming and going to perform too many different tasks. From the nurse's perspective, the problem with the factory model was that she never had a sense of a finished product— she felt like a factory worker.

It was not surprising that a new system came into being. *Team nursing* created a system in which nurses could have distinct products—patients of their own (somewhat like private duty). The patient would be served in his personhood, all his needs would be considered; he would no longer be a unit on an assembly line (nor would the nurse). All this would occur because the patient would be exposed to fewer workers who would know him better: his team.

With all its attempt to correct the flaws of functional nursing, team nursing did not escape the task delegation design of functional nursing. True, the team leader designated which team members would do which tasks rather than the head nurse; but that changed the leadership not the focus on task delegation. In building a team of members, a group who knew "their patients" intimately, the system tried to superimpose the *patient focus* of private duty on top of the *task focus* of functional nursing. Yet leadership decisions still were focused on which team member should do what.

Other flaws of team nursing related to the managerial and coordinating functions. Management had been pushed down the line from an experienced head nurse to a less-experienced team leader, a nurse not always comfortable delegating or managing people as a work team. Although fewer personnel saw every patient, the coordinating activities actually increased because several people (RN caregiver, nurse aide, RN team leader) might be involved with each patient without their roles and responsibilities being as clearly defined as in the old system. The team leader was daily deciding anew who would do what. Coordination problems with other groups also increased because team leaders tended to change from day to day, and physicians balked at never knowing with whom to discuss their patients' needs.

A few places tried to bandage the coordination problems by making more intimate groups. A miniature form of team nursing called *modular nursing* carved out even smaller teams—fewer nurses for fewer patients. This trend died quietly because it prevented flexible use of staff, and it offered nothing new because its basic structure was identical to that of team nursing.

The next system of care assignment, the antithesis of team, was *primary nursing*. It resolved the coordination and management problems of team nursing by a return to a patient-based, rather than task-based, work design. Namely, if a single nurse were responsible for a patient's care, then coordinating and assigning problems would be at a minimum. Primary nursing (often accompanied by RN professional staffing) owed its existence to the economics of the health care environment of the time. Institutions were hiring more professional nurses and fewer licensed practical nurses and nurses' aides for several reasons. First, most insurance reimbursement systems paid costs incurred without questioning them. Second, nonprofessional staff, through active unionization, had received substantial salary increases. Suddenly the RN, who knew more and could do more, became cheap at the price.

In times when nurses earn comparatively low wages and there is no critical shortage of them, nurses are not treated as important resources. Nurses tend to have a good work ethic and be self-monitoring, so it pays to use them as all-purpose workers if they are not costly. The trend of professional staffing (along with primary nursing) pushed this strategy to the hilt and was successful as long as nurses were plentiful and their wages suppressed.

The argument for primary nursing went this way: If only one nurse were responsible for each patient, and she was educationally prepared to complete all his care needs, then coordination needs would fall away and patients would get the best, individualized care. In effect, we were back to private duty, the chief difference being that the primary nurse now had more than one patient.

The flaw in the primary nursing model became evident rather

quickly. The primary nurse was present on the care unit for only 40 or fewer hours of 158 hours per week. The realities of the situation forced the primary nursing model to shift from a care *delivery* model to a care *planning* and *accountability* model. Actual care duties fell to others in the absence of the primary nurse and sometimes even in her presence if she had a heavy case load.

TODAY'S PRACTICE ENVIRONMENT

We were about at that stage when today's nursing shortage (at first a shortage in available nurses, then a shortage in the number of nurses an institution could afford to hire) created a demand for change. Salaries rose, and it no longer made sense for employees to pay high hourly rates for professional personnel doing lower level tasks. Enter once more a functional type of nursing, in this case, restructured practice. More economy and efficiency were needed; fewer nurses would need to achieve more. Such circumstances always require a task orientation, and restructured (re-engineered) practice returns to the task orientation of team nursing and functional nursing. The principle is the same: division of tasks.

Despite its task orientation, restructured practice retains some of the patient focus of the primary system by keeping the planning and accountability function centered in a single nurse for each patient, the case manager. In this sense, restructured practice models of today blend the two foci—the patient and the task. Figure 18-1 shows the rise and fall of historical assignment systems between the two parameters of a patient focus and a task focus.

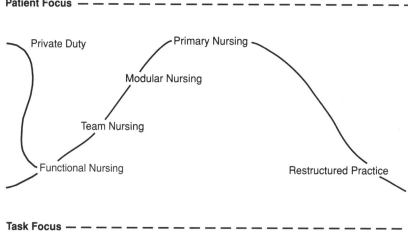

Patient Focus —

Private Duty

Primary Nursing

Modular Nursing

Team Nursing

Functional Nursing

Restructured Practice

Task Focus —

Figure 18-1.   *Care delivery models on dimensions of patient and task focus.*

The elements that drive our assignment systems can be seen through the theoretical model provided by Drucker (1974, pp. 551–557). He claims that all work is designed around one of four motifs—(1) work and task, (2) relations, (3) results and performance, and (4) decisions. Drucker's design logics (as he calls them) compare to Aristotle's formal, final, material, and efficient causes. Decisions start the process, that is, they are the efficient cause of management; work and task are the material causes; results and performance represent the final cause; and relations comprise the formal cause.

Restructured practice rests solidly in the design logic of work and task, but never before have we had a system that looks at all four of Drucker's design logics simultaneously in such a dramatic way. The design logic of *work and task* predominates because the restructuring involves a comprehensive look at what needs to be *done*, that is, the nitty-gritty tasks. Yet, more than in any prior system, what needs to be done is determined by the desired *results and performance*. (Hence, the introduction of case trajectory paths monitored by case managers with their eyes continuously on outcome goals.) As Sommerville (1996) said of her head nurse function, the kinds of questions she asks staff changed. With the outcomes orientation, she asks, "Where are your patients in relation to the outcomes you expect to achieve today? What should be happening? What is actually happening? What, if anything, can be done about it and by whom?" (p. 85).

More than in any prior system, the question of who will do what (*relations*) is open for revision. Extensive role examination and redefinition is the rule under restructured practice. Finally, there is intensive work concerning what *decisions* (and what sort of decisions) can be made by the various levels of worker, with a great downward shift in decision power occurring. Although it is conceptually separate from restructured practice, revised practice is often coupled with another decision-based system: that of self-governance in which nursing units or departments function with autonomous decision-making. Although each model differs, the notion is that nurses should be responsible for their own practice, which involves making and being accountable for the major decisions that affect their work life. Rose and Reynolds (1995), in reporting on the Johns Hopkins Professional Practice Model (PPM), explain:

> *Decisions should be made closest to where the outcome will be felt, so that participants have a sense of ownership for the change. (p. 2)*

No nursing unit, however, is entirely free of overall administrative authority, but the amount of autonomy can be extended greatly over past practices. As Rose and Reynolds (1995) say:

> *The scope of autonomy needs to be established and agreed on before the inception of any PPM. Mapping the boundaries of authority and control will foster trust between nursing administration and the nurses on the unit. (p. 2)*

Where self-governance is in place with restructured practice, another thread from Drucker's design logics (ie, decisions) is in place. Although the balance of the system focuses on tasks (nuts and bolts), restructured practice is the closest we have ever come to a system balancing on several design logics simultaneously.

REDESIGNING ROLES

Redesigning roles is the crux of the new system, with assignments made on the basis of the qualifications of the people who will do the tasks. The higher the preparation, the more complex the tasks. The principle is one of safeguarding precious resources—in this case (as in functional nursing) the resource of professional nursing time.

The modes of restructured practice are diverse, interesting, and even—some would say—exciting. One of the most interesting things is the way the pie is being sliced. In the old functional system, every institution sliced the pie identically. Everyone had a medicine nurse, a treatment nurse, and so forth. In restructured practice, each institution makes its own divisions—and the pies are being carved in all sorts of creative patterns. Restructured practice relies heavily on specialists, each doing his unique job.

Nor is all of today's specialism related to clinical phenomena. Role differences are crucial to what people do in the new systems. The two newest professional roles are that of the case manager and the nurse practitioner. Yet the greatest innovation has been in the growth of new types of technicians. These technicians can perform anything from limited nurses' aides tasks to highly technologic procedures. The generic term used for all these workers, from aides to technicians, is *unlicensed assistive personnel* (UAPs).

When one looks at restructured practice as it affects RN roles, the least common sort of restructuring concerns differentiating what 2-year and 3-year nurses do from what a 4-year nurse does. This change, the one most hoped for by nurses from academia, was the least prevalent because it set limits on the flexible use of nurses. More typical is differentiated practice between an RN and a technician. Some places, with RN–technician teams or RN–LPN teams, use a variant of Manthey's (1988) paired-partners concept.

In the paired-partners concept, an RN has a permanent partner, an LPN or nursing assistant/technician, who invariably works with her. In places where the luxury exists, the linkage is a function of the senior nurse selecting her own partner. In the idealized form of this practice, the permanent work team shares the same duty schedule. Other places use the term paired-partners more loosely, meaning two people who are assigned to work together on a given day.

In the more contained concept, the union is lasting, and the RN is able to train the lower level worker in what she wants done and how she wants it performed. In this way, tasks move to the lowest level, and tasks once seen as higher are done by lower level personnel properly taught and supervised.

Another growing application of differentiated practice and paired partners, involves paired physicians and RNs. Sometimes this is called the advanced practice model. In the advanced practice model, the nurse member may function quite independently, with protocols negotiated and signed by her physician partner. One sees this sort of practice most often where nurse practitioners (rather than clinical specialists) are teamed with physicians, for example, acute care nurse practitioners in emergency room practice. Ironically, the latest trend is for the RN partner-practitioner to replace her acute care physician colleague because of a shift in federal funding strategies.

The other major role change for the RN was the new role of case manager. This role uses Drucker's design logic of performance and results because it focuses directly on managing patient care outcomes for a group of patients. The task of the case manager is aided by the development of case maps with precise expectations for each day of hospitalization for each patient with a given condition. Nursing has developed great skill in producing these documents, and they have been publicized liberally (Blancett & Flarey, 1996; Cohen & Cesta, 1997; Flarey & Blancett, 1996).

In the best of models, restructured practice extends beyond the nursing division, examining anew all the role functions of the institution. When new roles are carved out, they may cross old departmental lines. For example, a function once done by nurses may be shifted to laboratory workers, or erstwhile intern functions in the surgical suite may be shifted to an operating room technician. The broader the scope of roles considered, the more efficiency can be achieved by a reordering of tasks and roles.

Restructured practice is characterized by diversity, experimentation, decentralization to the lowest level, recognition of specialism, and openness to the idiosyncrasies of both an institution and its practice environment.

SUMMARY

Restructured practice is the newest assignment system in acute care nursing. The method is a reversion to a task orientation. In general, nurses prefer the opposite pole of the continuum, the patient focus. When a shift is experienced toward the task orientation end of the polarity, it almost always indicates the press of environmental circumstances, which has been the case today. The health care system is in the midst of adjusting its staffing mix. The answer to date has been that if nurses are paid more, they must expect to be fewer in number.

Because the restructured practice model involves more of Drucker's design logics than any previous model, the arrangements are complex. The introduction of a case manager role (results oriented) has altered the management model from a hierarchical one (head nurse exclusively in charge) to a matrix design. The head nurse (by whatever title) represents one authority line, whereas the case manager represents another. The staff nurse is accountable to both authorities for her care. Although a matrix is an interesting managerial form, it always takes more maintenance work than does the hierarchical model. See, for example, the descriptions of the complex relations involved in two such systems (Bunkers, 1992; Larson, 1992; Tonges, 1989a, 1989b).

Although restructured practice began in acute care, one can see elements of it in long-term care and other step-down delivery systems as they, too, cope with the same environmental stresses and scarcities. Restructured practice, though not an ideal system, is probably as good a response to a difficult environment as could be made by the profession in these times. It is the most complex assignment system in nursing's history.

REFERENCES

Blancett, S. S., & Flarey, D. L. (1996). *Case studies in nursing care management: Health care delivery in a world of managed care.* Gaithersburg, MD: Aspen.

Bunkers, S. S. (1992, February). The healing web: A transformative model for nursing. *Nursing & Health Care, 2,* 68–73.

Cohen, E. L., & Cesta, T. G. (1997). *Nursing case management: From concept to evaluation* (2nd ed.). St. Louis: Mosby-Year Book.

Drucker, P. F. (1974). *Management: Tasks, responsibilities, practices.* New York: Harper & Row.

Dunham-Taylor, J., Marquette, P., & Pinczuk, J. Z. (1996, March). Surviving capitation. *American Journal of Nursing, 3,* 26–30.

Flarey, D. L., & Blancett, S. S. (1996). *Handbook of nursing case management:*

Health care delivery in a world of managed care. Gaithersburg, MD: Aspen.

Larson, J. (1992, May). The healing web—A transformative model: Part II. *Nursing & Health Care, 5,* 246–252.

Manthey, M. (1988, March). Primary practice partners: A nurse extender system. *Nursing Management, 3,* 58–59.

Rose, M. D., & Reynolds, B. M. (1995). How to make professional practice models work. *Critical Care Nursing Quarterly, 3,* 1–6.

Sommerville, J. G. (1996, June). Outcome-based practice: Convince me! *Seminars for Nurse Managers, 2,* 84–85.

Tonges, M. C. (1989a, July/August). Redesigning hospital nursing practice: The professionally advanced care team (ProACT) model, Part 1. *Journal of Nursing Administration, 7,* 31–38.

Tonges, M. C. (1989b, September). Redesigning hospital nursing practice: The professionally advanced care team (ProACT) model, Part 2. *Journal of Nursing Administration, 9,* 19–22.

19 *Nursing Theory and Nursing Education*

Nursing education is presently undergoing a period of upheaval and change, both in general nurse preparation and in specialty education. Unfortunately, much of the change is not theory driven so much as a response to things happening in the health care environment. After the fact, theory is being evolved to reflect the changes.

CHANGES IN BASIC PREPARATION

Several major thrusts have changed the nature of basic nursing preparation in recent years. First is the shift toward including both acute and distributive care in the curriculum; second is the tendency to view master's level, rather than baccalaureate education, as the entry level for practice. Finally, a tension has arisen between the curricula that focus on high technology/pathophysiology versus those that focus on a holistic concept of nursing. This same pattern may be found in graduate education.

Acute and Distributive Care Models

In 1981, Lysaught (1981, p. 44) recommended that nursing should no longer incorporate all its content in a single curriculum; he recommended two tracks with separate licensure: the episodic (acute care) and the distributive (nonacute) models. That report was never adopted by the nursing community, and acute care remained the core of basic nursing education. Now, almost 20 years later, we find the distributive component being added to basic curricula everywhere—not Lysaught's plan of "either/or" but both. Part of the impetus for this is the change in the health care delivery system, that is, initiatives moving much patient care out of the acute care hospital and into facilities such as ambulatory and intermediate care facilities and home care. For many educators and practitioners, this represents the future of nursing. Others find themselves following the change simply because it is difficult to get student placements in acute care facilities as these facilities retrench and eliminate beds.

Presently, the Kellogg Foundation's Community Health Education, Research, and Service project sponsors various schools endeavoring to put distributive health care into their curricula. Matteson (1995) describes the Northeastern University experience. She tells what processes were followed to make the community linkages, what courses were created, and what changes were necessary from the old curriculum to the new one. There is not, however, an effort to capture the conceptual framework underlying the program. In contrast, Lysaught (1981, p. 44) proposed a curriculum based on three intersecting dimensions: (1) nursing behaviors (assessment, intervention, instruction), (2) patient condition (well, unwell, acutely unwell), and (3) environmental setting (distributive, episodic).

Master's Level Preparation as the Beginning Education Goal

Although the few early attempts to make the doctoral level the entry point for nursing never caught on, the popularity of the master's level as an entry point is growing. Many prototype programs admit students directly to master's work, often second career students already holding nonnursing degrees. The latter students often go into accelerated master's programs. Columbia University School of Nursing is a good example of this sort of accelerated program. Most programs of this type have had pragmatic success, attracting students who already have developed maturity, learning skills, and prior life successes. Beginning at a master's level suits these older students, who want fast-track careers as well as fast-track education. The master's prepared nurses fare better in today's job competition.

Some accelerated master's programs still prepare generalist nurses, but most (including the Columbia program) prepare specialists. Even though the enrolled students will earn a bachelor's degree and the appropriate credentials to sit for state board examinations along the way, the fact that this is not a program goal allows for a more streamlined progression into study of the selected master's specialty. Program models differ widely as to their content and rationales.

Technology/Pathophysiology Models versus Holistic Care Models

Master's programs also reflect the polarity between holistic and pathophysiologically based curricula. Because of state board examination requirements, holistic programs are unlikely to make their entrance at the baccalaureate level. Whole curricula have now been designed for these holistic programs, as for example, Dossey's (1997) core curriculum. The debate between these two philosophies is still the "hottest" issue in nursing theory. The growth in holistic theories and holistic programs has outpaced that of the pathophysiology models, but they started far behind.

Most nursing practitioner programs, not surprisingly, opt for the pathophysiology models. These are most compatible for physician collaboration and certainly are advantageous in circumstances where physicians are teachers in the program. However, many schools have a master's option that prepares students exclusively in holistic nursing (eg, programs at the University of Colorado and the College of New Rochelle, New York).

THE DISCIPLINE MODEL

Nursing theory informs a nursing curriculum whether faculty recognize it or not; a nursing curriculum conveys a theory (or theories) of nursing by virtue of the content selected. The discipline model may be a specific nursing theory adopted (or adapted) from a given nurse theorist; it may be a model designed by the faculty; or it may be an intuited image of nursing. If the latter, the intuition may be shared among faculty, or individual faculty members may have differing and competing images of nursing, bringing more than one discipline model into the curriculum.

The discipline model may be purposely brought to the foreground of the student's consciousness, or it may be unstated and assumed (perhaps not even clear to the faculty). When faculty members perceive nursing differently, the student may be exposed to different images of nursing in different courses and clinical experiences within a single curriculum.

Consideration of a discipline model raises many questions: (1) Need the faculty be aware of the model(s) dominant in its teaching? Is it necessary to for the student to recognize a model to learn its use? (2) Should the discipline model(s) be made evident to the student? Or is a model adequately conveyed by the curriculum content selected under its auspices? (3) Should a single discipline model be selected for a given curriculum? Or should multiple models be allowed to co-exist?

One or Many Discipline Models?

Having only one discipline model in a nursing program has several advantages. First, it enables a faculty to better organize and select learning experiences. Further, the model can serve as a criterion for evaluating student achievement. When a single model is the focus of group attention, its flaws are more likely to be corrected; it is more likely to be refined than when alternate models are used. However, when each faculty member selects the nursing model of her choice, she may have more zest for teaching. Sophisticated students may enjoy seeing how diverse models function, whereas others may be confused by the shifting images and approaches.

A beginning student will have more difficulty adjusting to disparate models than will a more experienced student. Use of a single model enables the new student to integrate knowledge from diverse areas of study and facilitates her induction into the nursing milieu. Use of a single model as the basis for a given first-level program does not preclude introducing the student to the fact that other nursing models exist. Indeed, it will help the student to understand the discipline model if she has other models with which to compare it. The other models, however, become informational content rather than models to be used in the student's practice.

At the graduate level of nursing education, students should be sensitized to the effects of diverse models on nursing practice. Here faculty have an obligation to make the student aware of multiple nursing models. Faculty may choose to do this by using two or more nursing models within the curriculum or, again, by using a single discipline model for the graduate program while introducing the student to other models as informational content. Often in master's education, different study options in the same school use different nursing models. For example, a psychiatric nursing program and a medical-surgical program are not likely to select the same nursing model for advanced education. Nor is a clinical specialist curriculum likely to use the same model as a nurse practitioner curriculum.

CURRICULUM MODEL

The curriculum model is the vehicle whereby the student is systematically introduced to the discipline models that dominates the program of study. The curriculum model distributes the content of a curriculum. Suppose, for example, that the faculty of a four-semester associate degree program elected to use Levine's (1971) theory of nursing as the discipline model in its program. Suppose, also, that for the curriculum model, Levine's four principles of conservation were selected, each as the basis for a single semester of study. In this case, the curriculum model and the discipline model would correspond.

An alternate approach would be one in which the content of the semesters was decided on a different principle (eg, on the distribution of materials along a health–illness continuum) with Levine's principles (all four of them) being applied internally in each semester. Levine's theory is still the discipline model, but the curriculum model no longer replicates the discipline model; it now contains another organizing principle: the health–illness continuum.

The curriculum model should facilitate learning of the discipline model if a single model has been selected. However, learning may or may not be improved when the curriculum model coincides with the discipline model. In the previous illustration, one might argue that the second curricular arrangement gives the student a better understanding of Levine's theory because all four conservation principles may be applied to every patient studied. In this instance, the curriculum model that differed from the discipline model better facilitated learning than did the direct application of the discipline model. Often a curriculum model deviates from the discipline model to support learning theory. Also, some nursing theories simply are not formulated in a manner that provides for the distribution of curriculum elements. In these cases, the nursing theory will be subordinated to other organizing themes. The critical factor is that all organizing themes (primary and secondary) be compatible with each other.

Nursing Departments as the Basis of the Curriculum Model

When a faculty does not want to be limited to a single discipline model, a common practice is to use specialty departments as the primary organizing principles of the curriculum model. This produces a curriculum model with segments of the following sort: fundamentals of nursing, medical-surgical nursing, obstetrics, pediatrics, psychiatric nursing, and public health nursing (assuming the school has the traditional departments). These six blocks of study could be used to organize a baccalaureate program, with the student moving from one segment to another sequentially. The vulnerability of a curriculum organized by departments is that the content tends to have little interplay within the curriculum because each area is self-contained and based on a different set of premises, for example:

Area of Study—Underlying Premise
- Fundamental of nursing—skills (behavior-based)
- Medical-surgical nursing—body systems-based
- Obstetric nursing–life event-based
- Pediatric nursing—life phase-based
- Psychiatric nursing—patient behavior-based
- Public health nursing—epidemiology-based

With the department-driven curriculum model, every major block of study is derived from a different theoretical base. Take, for example, the first two areas. In fundamentals, the students learn that nursing is the performance of skilled acts. Then in medical-surgical nursing, the primary divisions of study are determined by illnesses grouped according to body systems—respiratory disease, cardiovascular disease, and so forth. In many ways, the student is starting at step one again, in finding out what nursing is. For every block of study, the student's previous concepts of nursing will require revision; building on previous learning will be difficult. Each block of study will contain its own, unique programming for how one goes about nursing. The disadvantage of such an approach is that student learning may be slower; integration across course lines will not come easily. The advantage is that each block of study uses those theories that best fit with its subject matter.

Core Curriculum

Where traditional departments form the curriculum model, attempts at unity often involve a search for a *core* (shared notions or principles). It is presumed that this core can be taught first, unifying the diverse specialties. The argument usually fails because the meaning of core concepts (eg, *stress*) changes when applied in different contexts, for example, (1) the patient in labor, (2) the community undergoing gentrification, (3) the patient in anaphylactic shock, and (4) the patient experiencing a life crisis. The instantiations are so different that prior generalized knowledge (of stress, in our example) is meaningless; the applications are so unique that the concept must be relearned in each instance. If the notion of core applies at all, it should be a final synthesis, a capstone course, rather than an initial generalization.

BUILDING A CURRICULUM MODEL

When the departmental structure is not used as the basis of the curriculum model, many alternatives may be used to organize an educational program. One source, the components of a discipline model, already has been mentioned. For example, one might organize an eight-component basic program around Johnson's (1980) behavioral subsystems: (1) affiliation, (2) aggression, (3) dependency, (4) achievement, (5) ingestion, (6) elimination, (7) sex, and (8) restoration. Numerous schemes may be used to parcel out the curriculum:

1. Skills and techniques
2. Body systems or diseases
3. Life events—developmental, crisis, other
4. Life phases—birth to death
5. Patient behaviors
6. Locus of practice—environmental, institutional
7. Steps of the nursing process—assessment, diagnosis, planning, intervention, evaluation
8. Nursing goals—prevention, restoration, and sustenance

Peplau (1965) identified 10 organizing themes for curricula that still hold today: (1) area of practice, (2) organs and bodily systems, (3) age of client, (4) degrees of illness, (5) length of illness, (6) nurse activities, (7) fields of knowledge, (8) subroles of the work role of the staff nurse, (9) professional goal, and (10) clinical services.

Few curricula are organized along a single dimension. More often, two or three organizing themes are crosshatched to build a curriculum grid. Table 19-1 illustrates a curriculum in which selected *patient problems* form primary organizing threads. A second organizing theme, *life phases*, has been woven through the selected problems. In this curriculum, courses might be organized around patient problems or reversed and organized around life phases. In Table 19-2, another curriculum model interweaves the organizing themes of the traditional *body systems* and the *nursing process*. Not all themes are compatible with each other. It is not logical, for example, to have two contradictory processes (eg, nursing process *and* problem-solving) in a single model.

Every nursing education program should be able to identify the discipline model(s) and curriculum model that underlie the content of the program. Where consistency is sought in a curriculum, these structural aspects provide the matrix for it. Where diversity is allowed, it is even more important that students recognize the different ideologies and shifts in the meaning of nursing.

Table 19–1. *Curriculum Model Cross-Gridding Patient Problems and Life Phases*

Dominant Threads: Patient Problems

Secondary Threads: Life Phases	Problems of Oxygenation and Nutrition	Problems Related to Activities of Daily Living and Mobility	Problems of Fluid Balance and Elimination	Problems of Self-Image and Role Fulfillment	Problems of Pain and Discomfort
Infancy					
Childhood					
Adolescence					
Adulthood					
Senior citizen status					

Table 19–2. *Curriculum Model Cross-Gridding Body Systems and Nursing Process*

Dominant Threads: Body Systems

Secondary Threads: Steps of the Nursing Process	Skeletal System	Integumentary System	Circulatory System	Respiratory System	Alimentary System	Excretory System	Endocrine/ Reproductive System
Nursing assessment							
Nursing diagnosis							
Nursing care planning							
Nursing intervention							
Nursing evaluation							

CURRICULUM SEQUENCING

Whatever discipline model a faculty wishes to convey, they should do so in a manner that is educationally sound. Hence, an interplay necessarily occurs between theory of nursing and theory of education. A major design problem in a basic nursing curriculum model is the selection of the entry point and sequencing of content. It is difficult to introduce the novice to nursing because all its practice settings are rich in complexity and cannot be artificially simplified for the benefit of the learner. Even a "simple" patient interacts with a complex, unpredictable, and multidimensional environment. Because nursing situations are inherently rich and complex, it is difficult to know where to start.

Curriculum organization attempts to sequence in a way that is meaningful to the novice learner. Nursing is more than simply new knowledge content for a beginning student; it is a new milieu, a new role, a new world. The very complexity of nursing phenomena accounts for the stress that nursing educators place on the need for moving from *simple to complex* in organizing nursing curricula. Like many self-evident principles, the rule to move from simple to complex is easier to prescribe than to follow. Suppose a program moves from simple to complex by starting with a study of the cell, progressing to tissues (groups of cells), then to organs (groups of tissues), then to integrated systems (groups of organs), and finally, to the totally functional man (groups of integrated systems). This notion of simple to complex starts with simple building bricks (cells) and works toward more complex systems. However, what happens with this design is that the student studies hemolytic diseases and renal failures early in the program (cellular phenomena), heart failure later (organ impairment), and fractures of the extremities (integrated systems of the body) much later. The intended logic of simple to complex is confounded because hemolytic and renal cellular diseases are more complex than is heart failure (a mechanical problem), and the mechanics of heart failure are more complex than is the simple fracture (integrated systems of bone and muscle providing mobility). In addition, movement from cellular to integrated systems contradicts another educational principle: moving from the known to the unknown.

Suppose that the simple to complex dictate were to be applied in a curriculum with a life-phase focus. In this curriculum, the study of the ill child clearly should occur *later* than study of the ill adult because illness in a growing and developing organism is more complex than in a stabilized one. In this case, however, logical age sequence would dictate a different order: movement from birth to senescence. Again, the simple-to-complex dictate conflicts with another principle, in this case, the notion of logical sequence.

A third curriculum might move from wellness to progressively serious illness in an attempt to traverse from simple to complex. Yet one is reminded of Freud, who studied psychology in the ill rather than the well, because the maladies were more plainly evident in the extreme cases. Applying the dictate of simple to complex in moving from health to illness contradicts the educational principle of moving from the obvious to the more subtle. The self-evident needs of the ill may be simpler for the novice nurse to recognize and understand than are the more subtle health needs of the well. The application of educational prescriptions in nursing curriculum is not so simple as one might wish. In all three illustrations a single educational prescription (simple to complex) contradicted other principles.

LEARNING REQUIREMENTS

Because nursing is a practice profession, nursing education is education for action (praxis). What is learned in nursing can be grossly divided into three categories: (1) cognitive content, (2) psychomotor tasks, and (3) judicious application of both in the extant nursing setting. *Cognitive content* refers to all that information the nurse learns as background to her functioning (eg, anatomy, physiology, pathology, psychology, medical procedures, nursing techniques, and patient diagnoses). It is the knowledge she learns, not for its own sake, but so that she will have enough information with which to make accurate clinical judgments later.

Psychomotor tasks include those specific learned acts that nurses perform according to a given rationale by applying accepted techniques (eg, administering medications and treatments, implementing diagnostic procedures). Some of these acts are primarily mechanical although it may be difficult to separate the mechanical from the acts that require ongoing judgment to be made during implementation of the procedure.

The third sort of learning, *judicious application* of cognitive knowledge and psychomotor skills in extant settings, is more complex than the other two kinds of learning. This sort of learning clearly is the seat of independent nursing practice. It also represents the sort of knowledge that is most difficult to acquire and teach. To say it involves critical thinking skills is only the first step. Benner, Tanner, and Chesla's (1996) study of clinical judgment is an excellent guide for the sort of learning skills required here; it involves *recognizing* and *interpreting* phenomena and *adapting* care to the interpretations. As these authors point out, these skills do not come overnight:

- *The clinical judgment of experienced nurses resembles much more the engaged, practical reasoning first described by Aristotle, than the disengaged, scientific, or theoretical reasoning promoted by cognitive theorists and represented in the nursing process.*
- *Experienced nurses reach an understanding of a person's experience with an illness, and hence their response to it, not through abstract labeling such as nursing diagnoses, but rather through knowing the particular patient, his typical pattern of responses, his story and the way in which illness has constituted his story, and through advanced clinical knowledge, which is gained from experience with many persons in similar situations. This experientially gained clinical knowledge sensitizes the nurse to possible issues and concerns in particular situations. (p. 1)*

Studies such as this make us question nursing's tendency to shun any education that smacks of apprenticeship. This study indicates that immersion in clinical phenomena is the best path for meaningful learning.

TEACHING STRATEGIES

What teaching strategies are necessary to convey the required learning in nursing? The answers are simple for cognitive content and psychomotor skills. Cognitive content is easily transmitted through a variety of media: lectures, discussions, programmed learning, or reading assignments. For the average student, acquisition of cognitive content can be achieved in the absence of skilled teaching, provided an alternative information source, such as a good text, is available. Psychomotor skills require demonstration, return demonstration with corrective feedback, and skill development through practice. Few psychomotor skills of nursing are difficult although some, such as scrubbing in the operating room, require the learning of intricate, stylized behaviors. Even psychomotor skills become complex, however, when they must be modified according to a patient's response or altered physiology.

Learning to apply cognitive knowledge and psychomotor skills judiciously in the extant nursing setting is a complex learning task in which the nurse improves over time, learning from each clinical instance in which recognizing, interpreting, or adapting occurs. The major teaching effort in nursing should take place in clinical settings. Cases can be selected to allow the student to practice these skills, with the actual clinical cases preferable to written or audiovisual case studies.

Contrived case studies (simulations or written cases) may or may not teach clinical behaviors depending on their structures. Some instructors use nursing cases merely as devices to transmit normative, cognitive content. This happens when a typical patient is presented, and teaching his care follows the normative pattern. Such a case study is really a lecture in disguise. In an effective case study, the uniqueness and variations presented by a patient are the important factors. To teach the skills of recognizing, interpreting, and adapting, the important factor is not that the patient has a particular condition or problem, but that the case as presented is inconsistent, incomplete, miscast, or inadequately managed to achieve goals. The idiosyncrasies of the clinical patient inevitably intrude on a good study. Cases can be created that test important clinical thinking skills, but they take a lot of planning.

It is helpful if the thought process behind the teaching–learning strategy and the thought process used in nursing practice coincide. That way students can practice those thought patterns as they learn. A teaching strategy that uses one thought pattern cannot teach a student to use a different pattern. For example, a didactic lecture on the steps of problem-solving will not teach the student to problem-solve. Indeed, the teacher's behavior (1) identifies no problem, (2) uses no solution-seeking procedures, and (3) fails to present the subject matter as problematic.

We will examine briefly some teaching strategies that exemplify dialectic, logistic, problematic, and operational thought patterns. The appropriate thought pattern for students to learn in any given curriculum is dictated by the nature of the accepted discipline model, that is, the nursing theory used in the curriculum. In the classroom, correspondence will not occur unless it is planned for—but if it is planned for—the learning experience serves a dual function: teaching content and process at the same time.

Some teaching strategies are flexible enough to express more than one method. Lecture, for example, can be made to express any given thought mode simply by controlling the organization and plan of presentation. Some strategies are naturally good fits with specific methods of thought.

A Dialectic Teaching Strategy

The traditional dialectic teaching strategy is the dialogue or Socratic method. In dialogue, the teacher leads the student to develop and expand her own thoughts on a given subject, primarily by the use of well constructed questions and demonstrations of inconsistencies in, or contradictions to, the student's position. Dialogue proceeds through self-revelation, the student's insight being prodded by the teacher's use of added perspectives or challenges. In dialogue the student moves from a narrow conception of her subject matter to broader and more comprehensive understandings that encompass more events and more complexities. Contrary to popular usage, dialogue is not simply any conversational interchange; it is an interchange that assimilates new information into a synthesis with previous knowledge. Such synthesis is not merely additive in nature because the previously held knowledge itself is altered by the new information.

Logistic Teaching Strategies

A curriculum using the concept of mastery learning is logistic in design. This teaching strategy divides the components to be learned into an invariant learning sequence in which acquisition of Component A is a necessary prerequisite to acquisition of Component B, hence using a systems-building technique. Another logistic educational strategy is the use of programmed instruction. Linear programs feed the student clearly defined components of the knowledge system, one at a time, providing for reinforcement and testing of each component as the program progresses. As components are added and related to each other, the total knowledge system is amassed. More reliance is being placed on available self-instructional computer-assisted instruction these days, with large portions of many programs dependent on software. Most of these programs, including interactive audiovisual programs, follow a similar logistic system of assembling building blocks. Where branching logic is used, one can see the influence of an operational system instead.

Formative testing is a logistic teaching strategy in which the course is conceived of as consisting of separate and definite units. Tests are constructed to measure attainment for each given unit. Individually prescribed instruction is offered for those units in which the student fails to show the required mastery. Logistic teaching strategies demonstrate a concern with individual units and their interrelationships. When students learn patient care by following the case maps derived in case management programs, the system is similarly logistic. In logistic learning, elaborate systems may be constructed from the given components, but the focus is on learning the components and their relationships.

Problematic Teaching Strategies

A problematic teaching strategy involves the student actively in solving problems. The most common strategy is the use of the case study.

The case study focuses on the circumstances of a single patient, the objective being to organize that situation into one where the patient's problems are resolved. The case study method may be used sporadically or it may dominate the whole curriculum. The case study, more properly, the problem study, is a strategy that allows extensive manipulation on the part the teacher. For beginning students, she may identify the problems, letting the students seek solutions. Or she may use the case as a problem-seeking exercise, teaching students how to find the important factors among the array of available data.

Another variation in the problem study has to do, not with the presence or absence of components, but with the form in which the components arise. For example, presentation of the problem can vary on a continuum from a clear statement of the problem as given to a situation in which the student must search for and delimit the problem. The problem may be contained in a simple situation or a complex one. The problem itself may vary in its complexity. The condition of mind set also affects the level of difficulty of the problem. For example, if a student knows that a given case is being used in the study of defense mechanisms, she is likely to locate and define the defense mechanism with greater ease than she would in a case assigned in a different context.

The problem study also varies depending on whether it occurs in a natural or an attenuated environment. No written problem study displays an environment as complex as an actual patient case. Simulated patients come closer, but even they are scripted with limited information. Finally, the student might be given a real problem in an actual clinical case. The teacher can encourage problematic thought by the design of classroom lectures. Lecture material can be presented in the problematic mode, stating a problem and working through the steps to its solution. This gives students an opportunity to observe someone else using the problematic mode. Demonstrations also can be given, not as step-by-step procedures, but as the presentation of a problem and determination of various appropriate ways to solve it.

A problematic approach is a good fit in some nurse practitioner programs because the students must learn to diagnose and treat presenting problems. Because it fits the initial and subsequent client encounters, the choice of a problematic method is appropriate for such a program.

Operational Teaching Strategies

The operational mode focuses on the perspective of the agent. Debate typifies this mode by presenting opposing perspectives on the same topic. Similarly, a symposium uses speakers with different, though not necessarily opposing, perspectives on the same subject matter. Other operational forms focus on differences in the activities of the learner. Teaching by educational games is an example of contraposing activities. Such games are used in teaching nurse managers (though they are seldom adapted to clinical education). They involve actual moves and countermoves by opposing learners. The objective, as in the debate, is to defeat the opponent. Some educational games are played with human opponents; others have computerized opponents in the form of a program of moves and countermoves.

The in-basket exercise is a noncompetitive operational strategy used in the teaching of nurse managers. It may be contrasted with the problematic modes in the following way. Although the in-basket exercise may require problem-solving activity, the focus is not on a single problem and its definition and resolution. Instead, the focus is on a constellation of activities that may include solving problems as well as other actions, such as processing multiple pieces of information and selecting some items for attention while eliminating others. What is evaluated is not simply the adequacy of the solution for one or more selected problems, but the total performance— the whole sequence of varied activities on the part of the participant.

Operational thought, in the form of differential diagnosis, also is a method that may be useful in a nurse practitioner program. Indeed, it is the form most often used in medical education, and there is nothing wrong with exposing nurse practitioners to the same concept. Using a similar method does not rob them of their nursing orientation.

ISSUES THAT MAY AFFECT EDUCATION

The Pew Health Professions Commission (1995) claims that we need a 20% reduction in our training capacity for nurses, and this is threatening to many faculty who have built their schools in an era of sustained growth. Managing in retrenchment threatens faculty positions and school status within the home institution. Instead of planning for retrenchment, many schools increase their recruitment efforts, competing harder for a shrinking pool of applicants.

If one grants a school the right to compete irrespective of societal manpower projections, then one does not "begin at the beginning" in planning a program of nursing education; that is, the program will not flow from a societal need. Self-interest and survival tactics may lead a nursing program to create a special niche for marketing purposes or even to create a "need" not perceived previously in the community. The program that can define its difference is ahead of the game when the game is intensive competition.

If a marketplace perspective drives a program, the school must assess its educational rivals. What other schools in the area are perceived as vying for the same selected niche? If a competitor in the same schooling environment is better equipped to service this niche, the school might need to reassess and find another niche. Alternately, the school might decide how it could interest a different (new) population of prospective students.

One of the strategies taken today by vulnerable schools of nursing is to decrease their insularity. This involves organizing joint curricula or shared courses with other disciplines such as medicine, dentistry, and social work. Or it may involve joint work with a business school, a school of public health, or even with disciplines and departments with fewer obvious connections to nursing. Such expanded vision serves students well, while enabling the nursing department to conserve its shrinking resources and enhance its value to other departments.

Today, the greatest decision point for many schools occurs at the master's level when choosing which sort of advanced practitioners to prepare: clinical specialists or nurse practitioners. The decision has virtually been made in the job market and in prospective student preferences. On both counts, the practitioner role is ahead. This issue for many is whether to convert, whether to keep both specialist and practitioner tracks, whether to create a combined role, how to make appropriate curriculum revisions, and (where appropriate) how to recruit appropriate practitioner faculty. As happens when everyone gets on the same bandwagon, the issue of oversupply of practitioners looms on the horizon.

Another decision point involves determining the scope of a program. Will the school educate all levels from baccalaureate to doctoral? How many master's level specialties and which ones? Careful selection is replacing growth as the critical factor in school planning. The old system of doing everything for everyone does not play in today's environment.

Within virtually all basic programs, a major issue is how to convert from an acute care orientation to a comprehensive community care model. By whatever names, most curricula today are adding elements of ambulatory, convalescent, nonacute, chronic, and preventive educative care. The faculty must determine whether its courses will be "setting neutral" or designed around the diverse settings and types of care used in the program. Distributive education has certain challenges not faced in the episodic, acute care facility, primarily the fact that the student may not be exposed to as many patients, and there may be fewer available nurse role models. Sometimes this problem is mitigated if the faculty member has a private practice in the distributive facility. Nurse-run centers contribute to the solution of education in the distributive care world. Indeed, the joint faculty practice-teaching role has become the norm rather than the exception.

One method of coping with today's shifting health care demand is to organize a curriculum around processes rather than around the content aspects of the curriculum. Hence, today's curriculum may be heavy on tactics, strategies, so-called critical thinking skills, systems management, and processes of information acquisition and retrieval. Although this conversion to process orientation is a popular answer, pushed too far, it produces a curriculum that feels devoid of content.

Another factor affecting curriculum development today is the effects of an outcomes orientation in the marketplace. A focus on outcomes (the goal element in theory) demands more flexibility in one's approach to and choice of methods. Students no longer learn "the one right way" to do anything, and this means a complex and demanding curriculum, not to mention a sophisticated teacher.

Both today's outcomes orientation and the increasing reliance on quantitative data push the nursing faculty toward an orientation through looking at group norms for patients rather than the old focus on the patient's individuality. Reliance on case maps is fast becoming the norm in nursing practice, and faculty are likely to rely on these tools for clinical education of students. Although these maps may be adjusted on an individual basis, that is not the usual procedure. This is not to say that the individual patient gets lost, but that course content based on group data rather than individual outcomes has a different philosophy. The nursing student in such a program is taught to think in terms of group norms as a criterion for decision-making.

Another new (or returning) principle is the nursing focus on working with others to care for each patient. This viewpoint requires a more complex curriculum than an insular focus on the learner–patient interface alone because the student will require a good understanding of what each health care worker has to contribute to the joint effort. Focus on intra- and intergroup process may lead graduate programs to use curriculum elements of delegation and supervision, not to mention communication, negotiation, and other human relations processes. In the intra-, interprofessional approach, we need to consider whether our exclusive theories of nursing do us a service or disservice in our relationships with other players, especially physicians. Where outcomes are attributable to the combined work of many professionals, can each group approach the cooperative venture from a different theory?

SUMMARY

Nursing theory and nursing education intersect in many dimensions. Only a few elements have been discussed in this chapter. In today's nursing education, the changes tend to come first from environmental presses, with the rationale and theories to be developed later. An informed curriculum with thoughtful interface with theory and other curricular elements provides a coherent approach to educational design. Nursing education today, like case management, is dominated by (1) combined goals of quality and cost savings, (2) an outcomes orientation, (3) a group rather than an individual mentality, (4) an intra- and interprofessional approach to health care, (5) an expanding notion of the settings where care will be delivered, and (6) a consumer orientation (whether the consumer be patient or student).

REFERENCES

Benner, P., Tanner, C. A., & Chesla, C. A. (1996). *Expertise in nursing practice: Caring, clinical judgment, and ethics.* New York: Springer.

Dossey, B. M. (1997). *Core curriculum for holistic nursing.* Gaithersburg, MD: Aspen.

Johnson, D. E. (1980). Behavioral system model for nursing. In J. P. Riehl & C. Roy (Eds.), *Conceptual models for nursing practice* (2nd ed., pp. 207–216). New York: Appleton-Century-Crofts.

Levine, M. E. (1971, June). Holistic nursing. *Nursing Clinics of North America, 2,* 253–264.

Lysaught, J. P. (1981). *Action in affirmation: Toward an unambiguous profession of nursing: A longitudinal follow-up on the recommendations of the National Commission for the Study of Nursing and Nursing Education.* New York: McGraw-Hill.

Matteson, P. S. (1995). *Teaching nursing in the neighborhoods: The Northeastern University model.* New York: Springer.

Peplau, H. (1965, August). Specialization in professional nursing. *Nursing Science, 4,* 268–287.

Pew Health Professions Commissions. (1995). *Critical challenges: Revitalizing the health professions for the twenty-first century.* San Francisco, CA: Author.

20 *Theory, Research, and Knowledge*

Theory, research, and knowledge are intricately related to each other. They involve the knower, how he comes to know, what he knows, and the reality about which he knows. How one acquires knowledge (epistemology) is influenced by one's notion of reality (ontology) and what can or cannot be known about it. The sort of research recognized as valid in reaching conclusions determines the kinds of theory to which a nurse will give credence.

For example, if a nurse is a hard realist who believes that reality is "out there," unaffected by what is known about it, and that only entities that can be measured by empirical research truly exist, she is unlikely to accept a theory that includes the affect of the nurse as a major theory component. Nor will she rely on heuristic interpretation to give a theory meaning. Little agreement exists about what methods produce warranted knowledge or about what reality is like. Hence, it is easy to account for the plethora of nursing theories and approaches. A quick look at ontology (the nature of being or reality) reveals where the disagreements originate.

REALISM VERSUS CONCEPTUALISM

Two broadly opposing ontologies appear in nursing theory—realism and conceptualism—and the two approaches are irreconcilable. In realism, one believes that the world exists "out there," independent of the knower. Research seeks to discover and explain the nature of that external reality.

263

In conceptualism, reality is not independent of the knower. Invention, rather than discovery, is the dominant mode of knowing reality. Reality is a negotiation between the knower and the environment. In its ultimate form, solopsism, the knower is believed to be the sole creator of reality; it is a mental act within the mind of the knower.

Realism and conceptualism are the extreme poles, with all sorts of variations on the continuum between them. Any ontology has an impact on the kinds of nursing theories accepted as valid and on the methods selected for research.

Calling them scientific paradigms, Newman (1992) separates out three ontological positions that have particular pertinence to nursing. The first is the particulate-deterministic view, describing phenomena as, "isolatable, reducible entities having definable properties that can be measured" (p. 10). Newman's intermediate position, the interactive-integrative paradigm, "views reality as multidimensional and contextual. It acknowledges the importance of experience and includes both subjective and objective phenomena" (p. 11).

In her last category, the unitary-transformative, "the human being is viewed as unitary and evolving as a self-organizing field, embedded in a larger self-organizing field. . . . Knowledge is personal. . . . Inner reality depicts the reality of the whole" (p. 11). This last point moves toward what we have called solopsism because so much of reality is placed in the evolving human being.

These three spots on the continuum mark the basic world views under which most nursing theories can be classified.

RESEARCH AND THE NATURE OF REALITY

The diverse ontological positions all have their own methods for validating knowledge. Popper (1953), a philosopher who falls in the camp of the realists (or under Newman's particulate-determinist paradigm), makes the following link between a reality that is "out there" and the method of knowing it. Because all of reality is objective, Popper asserts, all research involves the same process. He holds social scientists to the same methodology as bench scientists (ie, to repeatable experiments to be confirmed or refuted by controlled replication studies):

> *The only course open to the social sciences is to forget all about the verbal fireworks and to tackle the practical problems of our time with the help of the theoretical methods which are fundamentally the same in all sciences. I mean the methods of trial and error, of inventing hypotheses which can be practically tested, and of submitting them to*

practical tests. A social technology is needed whose results can be tested by piecemeal social engineering. (p. 365)

Popper's philosophy of realism sees the world as given:

Scientific results are "relative" . . . only in so far as they are the results of a certain stage of scientific development and liable to be superseded in the course of scientific progress. But this does not mean that truth is "relative." If an assertion is true, it is true forever. (p. 364)

Popper's world fits most closely under what we call the scientific paradigm. There is a reality apart from those who know it, and the way to know it is prescribed by empirical hypothesis testing. In contrast, in Dewey's (1938) reality, the result has precedent over his method (problematic):

. . . we are able to contrast various kinds of inquiry that are in use or that have been used in respect to their economy and efficiency in reaching warranted conclusions. We know that some methods of inquiry are better than others in just the same way in which we know that some methods of surgery, farming, road-making, navigating or what-not are better than others. It does not follow in any of these cases that the "better" methods are ideally perfect, or that they are regulative or "normative" because of conformity to some absolute form. They are the methods which experience up to the present time shows to be the best methods available for achieving certain results. (p. 104)

For Dewey, inquiry is:

. . . the controlled or directed transformation of an indeterminate situation into one that is so determinate in its constituent distinctions and relations as to convert the elements of the original situation into a unified whole. (pp. 104–105)

This process occurs through an interaction between ideas and facts. (This would place Dewey in Newman's middle range, interactive-integrative paradigm.)

Some observed facts point to an idea that stands for a possible solution. This idea evokes more observations. Some of the newly observed facts link up with those previously observed and are such as to rule out other observed things with respect to their evidential function. The new order of facts suggests a modified idea (or hypothesis) which occasions new observations whose results again determines [sic] a new order of facts, and so on until the existing order is both unified and complete. (Dewey, p. 113)

Although Popper's scientific method seeks to find out about a reality separate from his inquiry into it, Dewey's reality is itself changed in the process of inquiry. Method and reality are not separate:

The transformation is existential and hence temporal. The precognitive unsettled situation can be settled only by modification of its constituents. Experimental operations change existing conditions. . . . Only execution of existential operations directed by an idea in which ratiocination terminates can bring about the re-ordering of environing conditions required to produce a settled and unified situation. (p. 118)

. . . knowledge is related to inquiry as a product to the operations by which it is produced. (p. 118)

For Dewey, the inquiry itself produces the reality; it is not something "out there," totally separate from the investigation. Reality is an interaction between inquirer and environment.

Bergson (1955), yet another philosopher, presents a third view of reality and methods of inquiry:

. . . philosophers, in spite of their apparent divergencies, agree in distinguishing two profoundly different ways of knowing a thing. The first implies that we move round the object; the second that we enter into it. The first depends on the point of view at which we are placed and on the symbols by which we express ourselves. The second neither depends on a point of view nor relies on any symbol. The first kind of knowledge may be said to stop at the relative; the second, in those cases where it is possible, to attain the absolute. (p. 21)

Bergson illustrates what is meant by absolute knowledge:

Were all the translations of a poem into all possible languages to add together their various shades of meaning and, correcting each other by a kind of mutual retouching, to give a more and more faithful image of the poem they translate, they would yet never succeed in rendering the inner meaning of the original. (pp. 22–23)

Bergson refers to intuitive knowing as intellectual sympathy. Obviously, this method of knowing is far different from the methods previously examined:

If there exists any means of possessing a reality absolutely instead of looking at it from outside points of view, of having the intuition instead of making the analysis; in short, of seizing it without any expression, translation, or symbolic representation—metaphysics is that means. Metaphysics, then, is the science which claims to dispense with symbols. (p. 24)

Bergson's reality is different from either Popper's or Dewey's:

This reality is mobility. Not things made, but things in the making, not self-maintaining states, but only changing states, exist. Rest is never more than apparent, or, rather, relative. The consciousness we have of our own self in its continual flux introduces us to the interior of a reality, on the model of which we must represent other realities. All reality, therefore, is tendency, if we agree to mean by tendency an incipient change of direction. (pp. 49–50)

Bergson's world is at the far end of the pole in conceptualism, reminding us of Newman's unitary-transformative world view. Here, then, three different world views require three different methods of inquiry or research. In each case, the acceptable method of research depends on the sort of reality assumed. The conception of reality dictates the nature of methods perceived as appropriate for the acquisition of knowledge.

Wilber (1996) provides yet another view of reality and the means of researching and validating it. He claims that there are three different world spaces, each dominated with its own objects and ways of knowing. These are the worlds of the senses, of the mind, and of the spirit. One knows the world of the senses, he says, by measurement. This involves empirically designed, quantitative replicable research. Consensus in this world is by scientists who all agree on and use the same methods of knowing.

The world of the mind, which deals with logic, ideas, and concepts, also produces verification by consensus, but the consensus is through the psychological and philosophical insights exercised by those trained to use the eye of mind. Similarly, the eye of spirit is validated by consensus among those who are trained in the rules of spirit, which involves direct, immediate knowing. In this case, the answer is a sort of mysticism, not associated with either measuring or insight. For Wilber, each world requires consensus but only from those trained to adequately use the method appropriate to the world under review.

> . . . *each of these modes of knowing has its own specific and quite valid set of referents:* sensibilis, intelligibilia, *and* transcendelia. *Thus, all three of these modes of knowing can be validated with similar degrees of confidence; and thus all three modes are perfectly valid types of knowledge. Accordingly, any attempt at a comprehensive and graceful understanding of the Kosmos will most definitely include all three types of knowing; and anything less comprehensive than that is gravely, gravely suspect on its own merits. (p. xiii)*

Wilber's theory of a tripartite world is interesting because many nursing theories propose that man is comprised of three parts: body, mind, and soul, corresponding to his "eyes" of the flesh, the mind, and the spirit. In terms of validation, Wilber makes an interesting point that none of his three worlds can be held to the standard of proof of a different world without making a category mistake. If philosophers try to "prove" the existence of God through reasoned arguments (eye of the mind), they cannot. Nor can logic, for example, be proved through inductive, scientific testing; nor, as Wilber says, does religious illumination reveal that water contains two hydrogen and one oxygen atom.

THEORY AND RESEARCH

Theory and research form a recycling chain in which theory directs research, research corrects theory, and corrected (or confirmed) theory directs more research. A theory cannot be subjected to direct testing. Instead, one reasons that: if Theory X is true, then Consequences Q, R, and S will follow under Conditions A and B. Through research, one tests whether these predicted consequences actually occur under Conditions A and B. If the predicted consequences hold up under rigorous research conditions, then the theory is confirmed.

Of course, someone else may always come along later with an equally logical (or better) explanation of why Consequences Q, R, and S occurred under Conditions A and B. Theories are not proven; they are confirmed. Confirmation (or validation) simply means that, no cases to the contrary, a theory is accepted as an explanation of a phenomenon until a better explanation comes along. Seekers after eternal truth had better not rely on the research–theory cycle.

What are the outcomes of research? One possible outcome is that an original theory may be disproved or require modification. Often the researcher is not so fortunate as to recognize why a theory did not work or how it must be modified. Nevertheless, a theory disproved is a positive research outcome because it eliminates one false lead.

In finding one theory invalid, a researcher may formulate an entirely new theory as she gains insight into the relationships among the variables under study. The new theory may itself suggest further nursing research. Any given research may: (1) confirm a theory, (2) disprove a theory, (3) suggest modifications to a theory, or (4) suggest development of an entirely new theory.

Some theories arise with a subject matter and method that make the testing formidable. Think, for example, of the medievalists who tried to find irrefutable proof for the existence of God. For other theories, the research that would constitute confirmation may be imagined, but impossible to perform. Much of the validation research Einstein conceptualized to support his theories was not possible until decades later, when appropriate measuring devices had been invented.

NURSING: TWO CAMPS

In nursing, theorists have often divided into two camps, one close to the positivist (realist) view, the other close to the conceptualist view. Each "side" has developed its own theory bases using very different methods of seeking knowledge.

The positivist view, driven by the classical experimental design, hypothesis testing, and what gets termed the scientific method (hard science, in other words) accepts only controls, quantitative procedures, and statistical manipulations. Experimental design may vary, of course, because in certain situations the variables simply cannot be manipulated. Retrospective analysis of data is one such variation. Whatever its design, the quantitative method looks at the component parts of the phenomena under study, seeking to describe the interrelationships among them. The objective is to create explanatory theory, and where possible, situation-producing theory.

The nurses closer to the conceptual understanding of reality often preferred qualitative research, using heuristic testing and various forms of phenomenology (what Wilber might label methods of the mind, not the senses).

For much of our history, nurse researchers at the pole labeled with notions of positivism, empiricism, or quantitative research opposed what they perceived as soft science and soft methods, in other words, subject matter that was not strictly objective and methods that were not quantitative. Eventually nursing reached a compromise position where both sorts of research and both world views were accepted as valid pursuits. The quantitative versus qualitative debate became an issue of preferences instead of right versus wrong. Now, ironically, some researchers on the qualitative end are trying to suppress quantitative research in nursing as they were once suppressed.

Qualitative studies (focused on subject matter conceived closer to the conceptualist end of the continuum) started off with phenomenology as the chief method of inquiry. So-called grounded research (becoming immersed in the phenomena under study) grew in popularity. That popularity continues until today, but we now have at least two popular versions of phenomenology, each with its own particular twist. To understand how hermeneutics and critical theory differ from each other and from phenomenology, let's look first at the original system.

PHENOMENOLOGY

Phenomenology, a method of inquiry frequently associated with existential and holistic theories, sees the inquirer's direct experience as a legitimate way of coming to know. An epistemology as well as a method of research, phenomenology asserts that things must be known in their entirety rather than by reduction to their parts. Phenomenology reinstates the primacy of the subjective qualities of the matter under study. It is a deliberate effort to set aside scientific interpretations that reduce an entity to component parts; it preserves the view of the subject matter as experienced by the inquirer.

Phenomenology maintains that experience and the thing to which it refers are inseparably linked. The method may be applied to an object or an abstraction; one can explore meteorites or concepts such as beauty or human anxiety. Phenomenology seeks to reveal a thing in all its dimensions, in all its richness. Wilber would call phenomenology a science of the mind, not a science of the senses. The phenomenological method holds that the inquirer's direct experience of a thing is the way of coming to know it; phenomenology is a belief system about how we come to know (epistemology) as well as a method of research. It asserts that things must be known in their entirety rather than by reduction to their parts. Knowing the parts is not enough to understand the thing in itself.

Limitations of the Method

When phenomenology is selected as the research method for inquiry into a human process like nursing, the terminology "grounded theory" is often applied. Both terms refer to the researcher's immersion in the domain under study. Although this method escapes some of the narrow limits of reductionistic research, it is not without its own limitations, chief among them, researcher bias. The researcher tries to control bias by "bracketing," an attempt to see the phenomenon under study anew, setting aside one's previous thoughts, perceptions, and experiences with it. The issue is to what degree people can remove themselves from ingrained ways of thinking, habitual prejudices, even societally dictated meanings to which they have been previously exposed.

The Method in the Method

How one goes about implementing a phenomenological approach is difficult to describe because it involves an individual sensitivity unique to each subject. The process involves serious immersion in one's subject matter, immersion with a will to see the phenomenon anew, to view it with fresh, unencumbered vision. Whether the subject is human beings or relationships between human beings (as is often the case in nursing), it involves studying the relationship (or the people) as they are experienced or as they themselves experience the phenomenon, that is, in context.

The researcher attempts to identify all the themes that emerge, remaining immersed in the subject matter until no new ones surface. These themes constitute the "findings" of phenomenological research; that is, they comprise descriptions that others may use to better understand the essence of the phenomenon. Or the themes may comprise the categories in which others eventually construct empirical research.

As a method, phenomenology has been closely associated with existentialism and holism. The fit of phenomenology with these contextual themes is easy to understand. Existentialism focuses exclusively on the human being—his actions, feelings, and being. Nursing's existential theories do the same thing. Like holism, phenomenology attempts to see its subject matter as a whole, that is, in its entirety.

HERMENEUTICS

Hermeneutics, a derivation of phenomenology, is still popular among nurse theorists. Hermeneutics interprets human phenomena not to uncover universal laws but to explicate context, producing understanding rather than knowledge of the subject under inquiry. Hermeneutics aims for agreed-on interpretation of the meaning of events taken in context. Rabinow and Sullivan (1987) describe the movement this way:

> *For the human sciences both the object of investigation–the web of language, symbol, and institutions that constitutes signification–and the tools by which investigation is carried out share inescapably in same pervasive context that is the human world. (p. 6)*

Interpretations begin, they say:

> *. . . from the postulate that the web of meaning constitutes human existence to such an extent that it cannot ever be meaningfully reduced to constitutively prior speech acts, dyadic relations, or any other predefined elements. (p. 6)*

Rabinow and Sullivan see meaning as being somewhere between the subjective minds of the actors and out there:

> *These meanings are intersubjective; they are not reducible to individual subjective psychological states, beliefs, or propositions. They are neither subjective nor objective but what lies behind both. (p. 7)*

They characterize hermeneutics as a system that:

> *. . . heighten(s) the contrast between knowledge seen as technical project . . . and knowledge seen, in the human sciences, as inescapably practical and historically situated. (p. 2)*
>
> *Holistic explanation in the new forms seek to organize a wide variety of human phenomena that cannot be comprehended through models based on linear relations among elements. (p. 5)*

Patterson (1991) criticizes hermeneutics because: (1) the criteria for judgment of interpretations are lacking, (2) there are political objections to interpretive social science, and (3) it fails the criterion for empirical social science.

CRITICAL SOCIAL THEORY

Critical theory or critical social theory is the next derivative method arising out of phenomenology. The goal of this method is to free the knower from the biases of societal ideologies. This variant is advocated in feminist theories that envision distortions arising from the false overlay of values and behaviors in a patriarchal society.

Although the notion of correcting distortions in perception is laudable, some theorists use the method to justify their own agenda, often that of advancing feminist doctrine. In other words, the researcher may be invited to exchange one interpretive lens for another.

RECAPITULATION

In general, the conceptual, qualitative positions on research contrast to the methods clustering around the realism polarity. Kim (1990, p. 2) defines the field of nursing research as cast on three philosophical paradigms: analytical empiricism, Heideggerian phenomenology, and critical social theory. These three points are not a bad summary of the popular positions today.

Ironically, we have completed a circle in nursing, with qualitative research and related holistic theories challenging quantitative approaches for the lead in nursing research. One reason that quantitative positions are disdained is that, for a long time, their strongest advocates followed a narrow form of logical positivism—long since moribund in philosophy where it arose. Jacox (1974), an early advocate of logical positivism (or the received view as it came to be known), later rescinded the limitations of this format. In the original cast, positivism was a rather simplistic, building-blocks, logistic formulation. Jacox (1974, p. 5) identified these rules of theory construction:

1. A period of specifying, defining, and classifying the concepts used in describing the phenomena of the field
2. Developing statements or propositions that propose how two or more concepts are related
3. Specifying how all of the propositions are related to each other in a systematic way

This model continued to be dominant in nursing for many years. In 1978, for example, Fawcett wrote:

A theory is defined as "a set of interrelated (concepts), definitions, and propositions that present a systematic view of phenomena by specifying relations among variables." An empirically tested theory is composed of concepts that are narrowly bounded, specific and explicitly interrelated. (p. 50)

None of this is to say that the logistic, building-blocks method of theory development is wrong; it simply means that the logistic system is only one way to formulate theory, among many. Webster, Jacox, and Baldwin (1984) admitted this in a later criticism of the received view:

In retrospect it can be seen that several basic assumptions underlying the tenets of the Received View are traceable to the seventeenth-century world view. These assumptions were so basic to Received View practice that they were seldom explicitly articulated; they are the presuppositions of Received View doctrines.

Among these assumptions is the seventeenth-century emphasis on independence and atomicity, or the primacy of parts in comparison with the wholes which can be formed with them. Another is that mathematics is the language of nature. From this belief the tenet that theories ought to be formalized is a direct sequence. (p. 28)

Overreliance on the logistic formulation of theories in nursing denigrated theories that were not logistic in form. Or worse, it caused theorists or their advocates to reinterpret their theories in a logistic format, causing distortions in otherwise interesting theories. The problem was that the holders of this perspective tried to sell it as the only right way. Nurses who protested were seen as "unscientific."

Whall (1989), incidentally, asserts that logical positivism did not have as much impact on nursing as is credited to it. To most of us, however, it seemed that nurses were held to this narrow, logistic, wisdom—borrowed from the field of philosophy—far too long. As philosopher Suppe (1990) estimates, ". . . books in other disciplines which transmit the work of one discipline to readership within another discipline, are likely to be 10 years behind the cutting edge" (p. 1). Suppe points out numerous theorists and ideas no longer topical in their own fields still holding sway in nursing. He cites Kuhn and Laudan as examples (p. 2), and, yes, logical positivism (p. 8).

The same case might be made presently for hermeneutics, already getting less attention in philosophy than in nursing. Nursing's greatest vulnerability may be its tendency to rely heavily on other disciplines for its structure and methods.

Suppe (1990, p. 18) notes the tendency in nursing to equate scientific method with logical positivism, thereby claiming it as reductionistic and incompatible with holistic theory.

He notes two identity sets functioning in nursing:

Natural science = the scientific method = reductionistic = logical
*   positivistic = quantitative*
Human sciences = humanistic = antireductionistic = phenomenologi-
*   cal = qualitative (p. 19)*

Suppe finds both sets of equations untenable:

Further, that positivistic account is built around two independent com-
ponents, the so-called Received View on Theories *(wherein theories are*
axiomatic deductive systems given a partial observational interpretation
via correspondence rules), and the reductionistic thesis *that all phenom-*
ena in principle can be explained in the most fundamental terms . . .
these are two independent theses about science. (p. 19)

*   The claim that logical positivism favors a quantitative approach is*
just false. For the Received View treats qualitative observational descrip-
tions as most basic and fundamental; indeed the origins of positivism's
Received View on Theories are in the problem how to erect quantitative
theories on such a qualitative basis, and the Received View never did
succeed in giving a fully satisfactory solution to the problem. Thus it is
absolutely false that there is any intrinsic connection between logical
positivism, the scientific method, and quantitative research techniques.
(p. 2)

Suppe separates phenomenology from qualitative methods, noting that descriptions for an entire sample population can be manipulated by quantitative statistical analyses. These historical attempts
to make global, unnecessary connections between diverse concepts
may account in part for the backlash against empirical research in
nursing.

    Gortner (1990) protests this unfair representation, saying about
the literature on the so-called science of caring:

In all but a few of these essays, science is cast against humanism and
hermeneutics; the latter is seen as providing true meaning for all human
endeavor including scientific work on humans and by humans. (p. 102)

Her argument is not that hermeneutics has no place in nursing,
but that its place is narrow, limited to certain nursing situations, and
that those situations do not comprise the totality of nursing. Her
argument is that *understanding* (the goal of hermeneutics) does not
replace *knowledge*—achieved by empirical research. As Gortner says:

Human science activities cannot rest only with increased understanding;
nor can that understanding be taken as the sole criterion for explanation
as Benner has proposed. Human patterns and regularities and perhaps
even "laws" characterize the human state and undergird the whole
enterprise of society and human life . . . it is argued here that explica-

tion is a necessary requirement of nursing science as a clinical and human science, and that eventually such explanations will guide nursing action as therapy. (p. 104)

Norbeck (1987) adds, "When we make room for new perspectives, we must be careful not to throw away what is still useful from previous perspectives" (p. 29). Nor is she naive in her view of empiricism:

One of the central challenges to the empiricist view, however, is that objective observation of human behavior, stripped from contextual meanings, is a violation of truth. . . . As an empiricist, I subscribe to the notion that there are observables "out there" that can be measured. (p. 29)

The issue raised between supporters of empiricism versus advocates of phenomenology is an issue of ontology, epistemology, and research methods as well. To state the extreme cases, some researchers will forever be dissatisfied with a method that does not objectify and isolate variables. Such researchers will never grant that phenomenological approaches can lead to knowledge. In contrast, many researchers with phenomenological methods hold that much of what is *true* is lost in the very act of objectifying and isolating parts.

When one method, principle, or interpretation is taken as unassailable, any theory based on alternate premises can be criticized from that position. Take for example, the Nursing Theory Conference Group's (1980) criticism of Rogers' theory from the logistic perspective:

Terms have not been sufficiently operationalized to provide for clear understanding. By operationalizing terms is meant the description of a set of physical procedures that must be carried out in order to assign to every case a value for the concept. For example, to operationalize the concept of width is to place a tool consisting of the units of inches or centimeters along the edge of the item to be measured and count the units.

Because of the lack of operational definitions, research done to support or verify the principles provides questionable results. (p. 90)

The criticism of Rogers is essentially that she is not using a logistic method. The eternal validity and correctness of the group's own method over Rogers's was never questioned.

Wilber's suggestion may give us the way out of this dualistic nursing dilemma. We can have research of the senses (empirical), research of the mind (various phenomenological methods) and even, for those nursing theories that add a spiritual component, research of the spirit (direct apprehension)—if we get so bold.

SUMMARY

Research methods and theory preferences change as notions of reality change, and, indeed, the theories and research methods may themselves inform the perspectives on reality. Whatever theory a nurse uses, she should understand the world view it represents as well as what research methods are appropriate, given its content and context. We would hope that nurses would develop a general respect for alternate views of other people, including the research methods appropriate to their world views.

REFERENCES

Bergson, H. (1955). *An introduction to metaphysics.* New York: Bobbs-Merrill.

Dewey, J. (1938). *Logic: The theory of inquiry.* New York: Henry Holt.

Fawcett, J. (1978, October). The relationship between theory and research: A double helix. *Advances in Nursing Science, 1,* 49–62.

Gortner, S. (1990, Spring). Nursing values and science: Toward a science philosophy. *Image, 2,* 101–105.

Jacox, A. (1974, January/February). Theory construction in nursing—An overview. *Nursing Research, 1,* 4–13.

Kim, H. S. (1990, September 8). *Identifying alternative linkages among philosophy, theory, and method in nursing science.* Paper presented at the Symposia on Knowledge Development, University of Rhode Island College of Nursing, Kingston, Rhode Island.

Newman, M. A. (1992, January/February). Prevailing paradigms in nursing. *Nursing Outlook, 1,* 10–13.

Norbeck, J. S. (1987, Spring). In defense of empiricism. *Image, 1,* 28–30.

Nursing Theories Conference Group (Julia B. George, Chairperson). (1980). *Nursing theories: The base for professional nursing practice.* Englewood Cliffs, NJ: Prentice-Hall.

Patterson, D. M. (1991, September 26). *Hermeneutics and the philosophy of praxis.* Paper presented at the Conference on Knowledge Development in Nursing, College of Nursing, University of Rhode Island College of Nursing, Kingston, Rhode Island.

Popper, K. R. (1953). The sociology of knowledge. In P. P. Wiener (Ed.), *Readings in philosophy of science* (pp. 357–366), New York: Charles Scribner's Sons.

Rabinow, P., & Sullivan, W. M. (1987). *Interpretive social science: A second look.* Berkeley, CA: University of California Press.

Suppe, F. (1990, September 7). *Knowledge development in the context of shifting world views: The philosophy-theory linkage.* Paper presented at the Symposia on Knowledge Development, University of Rhode Island College of Nursing, Kingston, Rhode Island.

Webster, G., Jacox, A., & Baldwin, B. (1984). Nursing theory and the ghost of the received view. In J. C. McCloskey & H. Grace (Eds.), *Current issues in nursing* (pp. 26–35). Boston: Blackwell Scientific.

Whall, A. L. (1989, Winter). The influence of logical positivism on nursing practice. *Image, 4,* 243–245.

Wilber, K. (1996). *Eye to eye: The quest for the new paradigm* (3rd ed.). Boston: Shambala.

21 *Advanced Nursing Practice: Implications for Theory*

Advanced nursing practice is the latest catchword in nursing, and it applies to both clinical nurse specialists (CNSs) and nurse practitioners (NPs), despite the fact that the roles have different goals and orientations. These roles have taken on more importance in recent years as the master's degree has become the gold standard for nurses. Many social and political events have brought about today's focus on the master's level of nursing practice, chief among them, shrinking employment opportunities for less prepared nurses—and, ironically, also fewer jobs for some better prepared nurses with doctorates. Equally important is the growing popularity of the NP role in the marketplace.

NURSE PRACTITIONERS

The NP movement started as a joint effort between nursing and medicine to prepare primary caregivers to handle uncomplicated patient cases. Midwives, anesthetists, and, somewhat later, pediatric NPs were early practitioner roles. The original practitioner programs taught selected nurses the elements of physical diagnosis and prescription, usually relying on a pathophysiologic theoretical model. Typically, the early programs were created outside of academia, often recognized by certification from professional specialty organizations. Later, the American Nurses Association (ANA) also joined the credentialing game.

Certification was offered as competition with academic credentials, moving us toward the British system. Now, most practitioners have both an academic master's degree and certification, with most certification programs requiring completion of a related master's degree before one sits for the examination.

With the growth in popularity of the practitioner movement, certification programs increased in number. Now most nurses have an "alphabet soup" of initials after their names. Common certificate programs include: certified nurse midwife (CNM), certified through the American College of Nurse Midwives; certified registered nurse anesthetist (CRNA), through the American Association of Nurse Anesthetists; pediatric nurse practitioner (PNP), through the National Certification Board of Pediatric Nurse Practitioners and Nurses or the ANA; critical care RN (CCRN), through the American Association of Critical Care Nurses; orthopedic nurse, certified (ONC), through the National Association of Orthopaedic Nurses; oncology certified nurse (OCN), through the Oncology Nursing Society; adult nurse practitioner (ANP) through the ANA or the American Academy of Nurse Practitioners; family nurse practitioner (FNP), through the ANA or the American Academy of Nurse Practitioners; geriatric nurse practitioner (GNP), through the ANA; neonatal nurse practitioner (NNP), through National Certification Corporation for Obstetric, Gynecologic and Neonatal Nursing Specialties; certified rehabilitation RN (CRRN), through the Association of Rehabilitation Nurses; and certified emergency nurse (CEN), through the Emergency Nurses Association.

Additional certification programs include (basic and advanced) nursing administration (CNA and CNAA), certified addictions RN (CARN), certified plastic surgery nurse (CPSN), certified correctional health professional (CCHP), certified enterostomal nurse (CETN), certified RN intravenous (CRNI), certificate in diabetes education (CDE), certified neuroscience RN (CNRN), and certified neurology nurse (CNN). Additional certifications are available in postanesthesia, for nurse–attorneys, for intravenous care, for mobile intensive care, for nutrition support, for occupational health, and others. Not all of the latter certificates are tied to academic credentials.

Still other certifications are in the planning, and the American Nurses Credentialing Center (ANCC) offers the general "certified" (C) and certified specialist (CS) for many specialties. The point is that we have become a profession of specialists, and many of the specialty certifications are closely linked to practitioner education, usually in academic, master's degree-granting programs.

Originally, NP programs were fought tooth and nail by many

nurse leaders who perceived the role to create "mini doctors" rather than "super nurses." It was easy for this fear to lodge because most of the early program teachers were physicians. The fear was that NPs would forget their origins and identify with the medical profession. Although this may have occurred in some early cases, it is clear that most NPs keep their nursing identity, and enjoy the "value added" from that orientation, namely, taking a more comprehensive view of the patient as a total person, not merely as someone with an illness or condition.

The practitioner role has grown because of its appeal to nurses, consumers, and insurers. Early in the movement's development, NPs filled positions suffering from a shortage of physicians. Subsequently, the practitioner roles, still highly tied to a sponsoring physician, created a new business model in which hiring physicians could expand their practices by hiring NPs and taking a percentage of the additional income produced by them. In this model, the more NPs, the greater the financial reward.

Today's financial reimbursement schemes have mitigated that situation, and many NPs are now reimbursed directly for their services. Today, the NP is more likely to be seen by the physician as competition in a field already made competitive by a physician oversupply. Insurers, however, have grown to appreciate the fiscal rationale for using NPs, and this ensures the continuance of the role.

Nor is finance the only recommendation for NPs to insurers. Indeed, the Columbia University School of Nursing, New York, has negotiated the first contract with an insurer (Oxford) in which NPs are reimbursed at the same rate as physicians. One case, however, does not yet make a pattern.

In a tight employment economy, the NP model offers more security to the nurse than other roles, albeit not a carefree ride, given the physician competition for jobs. Many nurses also like the idea of holding a job they see as more independent.

Carrino and Garfield (1995, p. 76) looked at the research on substitutability of NPs for physicians and found many studies that conclude the NPs provide care at a lower cost than physicians and provide care in areas where clients are not served by physicians. The authors identify and differentiate the practitioner role from the physician role, by NPs' emphasis on patient education, patient counseling, and more extensive verbal interactions with patients than their physician peers (p. 77). They also noted that most studies proved whatever they wished regarding the nurse role because nurse-designed and physician-designed studies measured different variables (those of prime importance to the profession doing the study) (pp. 78–79).

Practitioner Theory Models

Originally, with no adequate nursing theories for their extended practice, NPs often adopted the medical model. The use of this model still prevails today in many specialties. However, the development of practitioner specialties has created a need for both practitioner role-specific and practitioner specialty-specific theories. The work in this area is only beginning. The Shuler (1993a, p. 14) model for practitioners was one of the early models. Based on a wellness model and the nursing process, it claimed to advance a holistic approach to clients. The theory is presented in a protocol with hundreds of components beginning with the chief complaint/purpose of visit. This orientation would seem to negate the notions of wellness and holism. The authors hedge this point in their second article (1993b):

> NPs are therefore challenged to address the patient's response to potential and actual problems (nursing role), while assessing/treating the condition itself (medical role) when appropriate. (p. 73)

This description is a good example of today's models in that it adds a medical role onto a nursing role rather than attempting a synthesis. Campbell and coworkers (1995) also have a model that is additive, although it combines three elements: the CNS role, the extra NP tasks, and a conjunctive case management role:

> The advanced practice model we will describe consists of a blending of NP, CNS, and case manager roles in a collaborative practice model with staff physicians. (p. 176)

Ligas (1997, pp. 125–126), a physician and mentor, views the NP role as having several components: role adjustment, acquiring of cognitive material—of pathologies and physiologic mechanisms—and the need to develop problem-solving abilities when a problem does not fit into patterns stored in memory. He calls the latter task *reflection in action*. He pays particular attention to role transition, noting that in the past:

> . . . ultimately there was someone else—the patient's physician—who determined the course of care and assumed responsibility for outcomes . . . but now the nurse practitioner makes more unilateral decisions and is more responsible for good and bad outcomes. (p. 124)

He cites a problem that nurses have in adjusting to the added responsibility:

> *One of the most telling signs of an incomplete role transition is the attribution of decisions to others, and the use of what the sociologist Renee Anspach has termed the "agentless passive." (p. 124)*

Other authors recognize this pattern expressed in the excessive use of referrals by some NPs—referrals for situations that the NPs could have handled had they accepted the accountability.

We can expect work to continue in model development for the NP role. Much of the present work simply reflects tasks, that is, long lists of things the NP does for the client. I think the NP role will eventually be perceived primarily as a methods shift, with a move toward a problematic orientation (honoring the patient's presenting problem) or toward an operational system (using, like the physician, differential diagnosis).

CLINICAL SPECIALISTS

Clinical specialist roles tend to be discussed in terms of their clinical foci rather than in terms of role. In contrast to the discussions of the NP, CNSs are assumed to be directly involved in "regular" nursing care, albeit with the most complex cases. Because the CNS role is seen primarily as a traditional nursing role, many CNSs (and specialist programs) use the same theories as used in undergraduate education.

Nor is all theory the property of education programs; nurses in practice also are likely to explore the application of theory to specialty practice. McKenna, Parahoo, and Boore (1995a, 1995b) apply the Human Needs Model (HNM) to care of psychiatric patients in Ireland, finding that use of a nursing model improved perceptions of the ward atmosphere, patient satisfaction, staff views about nursing models, and patients' dependency levels. However, no significant changes were found in nurse satisfaction or in nurses' perception of patients' behaviors (1995a, p. 95). Some of the results of this study present problems because the authors purport to be testing the effect of applying "a nursing model," and this is never quite differentiated from the results of applying the HNM—the only nursing model tested.

This is not to say that all, or even many, specialized programs use nursing theories. Often specialty-related theory is drawn from other disciplines, for example, psychotherapeutic models, family and crisis theory, and pathophysiologic models.

Although most CNSs (and their educational programs) are still oriented toward acute care, we can anticipate that new clinical specialties will arise in distributive (nonacute care), and these will call for development of new nursing theories. McClung (1995, p. 69), in home health, for example, struggles to find a model for her practice. Identifying structure, process, and outcome as her commonplaces, she comes up with a model that includes payers, clients, home support systems, and home health agencies (structures); type and intensity of care interventions (process); and client and family satisfaction, quality of care, and cost effectiveness (outcomes). Some additional elements are included in each category, but the ones cited here are the primary concepts.

The CNS focused on clinical care has not fared so well as the NP in the employment market. Indeed, as nurse executives strive to keep up their staffing numbers in an age of retrenchment, they often sacrifice CNS roles for more of the less expensive staff nurses. Whether or not one agrees with this decision, the tactic is used.

Hence, it is not surprising that many CNSs seek out private practice. The CNS role is shifting, ever so gently, toward a more independent role, and many specialists today feel that their practice is every bit as independent as that of the NP, albeit located more directly in nursing. Use of nursing diagnoses, for example, may be seen as the equivalent of the diagnostic categories used by NPs.

Despite these moves toward independence, as a practical matter the NP role has won out over the clinical specialist role. One measure of this is the steady number of nursing education programs that have added NP programs or converted entirely from preparation of CNSs to education of NPs. Yet other schools have developed an amalgamated role, combining the strengths of both roles.

JOINT SPECIALIST/PRACTITIONER ROLES

The schism between the CNS and the NP still is a major theoretical debate in nursing (Bullough, 1992), but increasingly, the answer seems to be to accept both roles, or, more recently, to combine the two roles. The actual content of the CNS programs and their related NP programs (eg, a pediatric CNS and a pediatric NP) have become more similar than dissimilar in recent years. When Forbes, Rafson, Spross, and Kozlowski (1990) compared NP and CNS programs in gerontology and pediatrics, they found corresponding core requirements and minimal differences in content. As they noted, each curriculum has as its chief components the building of clinical judgment and leadership. Calkin (1984) also recognized the minor differences between the roles, with CNSs prepared for more indirect client services, whereas NPs were prepared for more direct service. This is not to say that all nurses, especially all educators, would agree with this position. To some degree, it may reflect the wide variance from one practitioner program to another as to quality and content. Many schools have converted to a so-called advanced practice curriculum that contains the best of both programs while preparing the graduate for certification as an NP.

SUMMARY

From a nursing theory perspective, master's education offers two challenges: (1) building nursing models to describe clinical specialty foci, and (2) building nursing models for both the CNS and NP roles— generic and specialty practice.

Specialty work is a ripe and promising arena for nursing theory development. Nor is it enough to create specialty nursing theories; they must be theories of adequate depth and precision so that our specialties develop as nursing fields and provide for interface with other professions whose work is closely associated with the nursing specialty. It is likely that theory development in the next decade will focus heavily on the advanced practice roles.

REFERENCES

Bullough, B. (1992). Alternative models for specialty nursing practice. *Nursing & Health Care, 5,* 254–259.

Calkin, J. D. (1984, January). A model for advanced nursing practice. *Journal of Nursing Administration, 1,* 24–30.

Campbell, M. K., Brandel, S. M., Daramola, O. I., Postallian, M. A., Dorris, G. A., & Provenzano, L. J. (1995). An advanced practice model: Inpatient collaborative practices. *Clinical Nurse Specialist, 3,* 175–179.

Carrino, G. E., & Garfield, R. (1995, Fall). The substitutability of nurse practitioners for physicians. *Nursing Leadership Forum, 3,* 76–83.

Forbes, K. E., Rafson, J., Spross, J. A., & Kozlowski, D. (1990). Clinical nurse specialist and nurse practitioner core curriculum survey results. *Nurse Practitioner, 4,* 43–48.

Ligas, J. R. (1997). Experience as preceptor to acute-care nurse practitioners students: One physician's view. *AACN Clinical Issues, 1,* 123–131.

McClung, R. L. (1995, January/February). Considerations for the use of a conceptual model in home health nursing. *Pediatric Nursing, 1,* 68–70.

McKenna, H. P., Parahoo, K. A., & Boore, J. R. P. (1995a). The evaluation of a nursing model for long-stay psychiatric patient care. Part 1—Literature review and methodology. *International Journal of Nursing Studies, 1,* 95–113.

McKenna, H. P., Parahoo, K. A., & Boore, J. R. P. (1995b). The evaluation of a nursing model for long-stay psychiatric patient care. Part 2—Presentation and discussion of findings. *International Journal of Nursing Studies, 1,* 79–94.

Shuler, P. A., & Davis, J. E. (1993a, January/February). The Shuler nurse practitioner practice model: A theoretical framework for nurse practitioner clinicians, educators, and researchers, Part 1. *Journal of the American Academy of Nurse Practitioners, 1,* 11–18.

Shuler, P. A., & Davis, J. E. (1993b, March/April). The Shuler nurse practitioner practice model: Clinical applications, Part 2. *Journal of the American Academy of Nurse Practitioners, 2,* 73–75.

BIBLIOGRAPHY

Watts, R. J. (1997). The critical-care nurse practitioner curriculum at the University of Pennsylvania: Update and revision. *AACN Clinical Issues, 1,* 116–122.

Index